# COINS FROM THE COUCH

# COINS FROM THE COUCH

### Tidbits from a Psychiatrist's Office

# Kay M. Shilling, M.D.

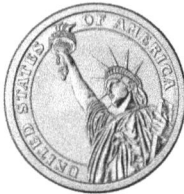

Wright Manor, LLC.,
Omaha, NE 68124

# Copyright © 2012

Layout in Georgia

First Edition, 2012 manufactured in USA
1 2 3 4 5 6 7 8 9 10 LSI 16 15 14 13 12


ISBN 978 0 615 71652 7


Wright Manor, LLC.,
Omaha, NE 68124

THIS BOOK IS DEDICATED
TO MY MOTHER

She persisted in inspiration,
guidance, courage, grace and fortitude.

20% OF ALL PROCEEDS FROM THIS
BOOK GO TO THE NON-PROFIT
ORGANIZATION

**Rosebud Foundation**

This organization provides at no charge
the materials and teaching for helping all
peoples learn knitting, crochet, tied edge
blankets and other craft arts when funding
to do so is not otherwise available.

**"Like" us on Facebook.**

# TABLE OF CONTENTS

CHAPTER ONE

Unique Psychiatry

Page 1


CHAPTER TWO

The Shilling Consistency System

Page 11


CHAPTER THREE

Medications

Page 41


CHAPTER FOUR

Caffeine, Alcohol, Pot, Etc.

Page 59


CHAPTER FIVE

Be the Barracuda

Page 71

CHAPTER SIX

Assertiveness Training

Page 79


CHAPTER SEVEN

The Care and Feeding of Women

Page 89


CHAPTER EIGHT

A Healthy Man

Page 103


CHAPTER NINE

Families

Page 109


CHAPTER TEN

Not Everything is Dementia

Page 139


CHAPTER ELEVEN

Don't Dismiss the Herbals

Page 157

CHAPTER TWELVE
Weight Loss Tips
Page 167

CHAPTER THIRTEEN
Educational Minutes
Page 183

Educational Minute #1
Post Holiday Blues
Page 185

Educational Minute #2
What is a Psychiatrist?
Page 187

Educational Minute #3
Two Types of Depression
Page 189

CHAPTER FOURTEEN
Articles
Page 191

Article #1
Holiday Blues
Page 195


Article #2
How to Help Stop the Shooters
Page 199


Article #3
Bible Only?
Page 205


Article #4
Humor is a Good Defense Mechanism
Page 209


Notes
Pages 214

# CHAPTER ONE

## Unique Psychiatry

---

**Coin #1:**
Psychiatrists do psychotherapy and
prescribe medications.

**Flip side:**
There are many unique approaches to
helping patients.

I decided to get right to it with a first chapter. I find that most of the time when people are seeking help or advice they aren't interested in waiting for it. This, I think, would include not wanting to wade through the usual book prefaces and introductions.

Psychiatry is a unique field of medicine that is often misunderstood. Movies and TV shows don't always help to depict what we really do as professionals or how we can really help. Sometimes, the "fear of the unknown" is what I hear the first time someone calls my office to make an appointment. The caller knows they are in emotional or psychiatric pain. If they have never been to a Psychiatrist or any other type of therapist they don't have a point of reference from which to draw or imagine what to expect, where to start, or where we start. Sometimes the discomfort I hear on the phone of the caller is someone who has been in treatment but has had a bad experience elsewhere and is unsure if my office will be different for them.

Psychiatry differentiates itself from other medical specialties in that there are different approaches to diagnoses, different approaches to psychotherapy, different theories and protocols to prescribing medications and just about as many of all of these as there are individual Psychiatrists.

I will present to you in this book what has been tried and true for me. I have been a doctor for more than thirty years. Along the way I have developed some methods and systems that have helped many patients in a variety of conditions.

This book is not to be a substitute for someone who needs the time honored actual treatment of a Psychiatrist. However, it might help do several things.

The tidbits or "coins" from this Psychiatrist's couch might be sufficient enough to help someone in a situational time of need. The tidbits or chapters may encourage someone to seek further help if they need it. The chapters and information could possibly enlighten or edify someone on their journey to understanding Psychiatry and what Psychiatrists do. The "coins" might help encourage change when change is needed or give someone a different perspective or give encouragement, support, or validation they previously were not able to have. Succinctly, I hope that the book and "coins" of my life's work to date will simply help someone, sometime.

This is what I do all day, every day that I am in the office. This book might be able to reach more people than what I can do one session at a time, 50 work weeks a year.

As I discussed above, each Psychiatrist

conducts their practice somewhat uniquely. I was trained to provide both psychotherapy and medication management, a combination that is currently somewhat unique to my practice. Many other Psychiatrists do just medication management appointments, but I like to do the psychotherapy as well. It affords my patients the opportunity to cover both at the same time and at the same place. When they choose this option they do not need to go to a separate appointment with a therapist at another time. I, also, though, like working with the patients who have other therapists and then I oversee their medication management only. In addition, there are those patients who prefer to have psychotherapy and no medications, but they like the psychotherapy to be performed by a Psychiatrist and not a therapist. I see these patients as well. What is important to share with you about all of this is that the "coins" in the book are derived from this unique aspect of practice.

I think it is important to add that I personally have a philosophy in my practice to minimize the use of medications wherever possible or practical. Just because I have the degree that allows me to prescribe, it does not mean that I think everyone needs or should be on medication that has symptoms. I very carefully evaluate a patient before I ever suggest a medication for any condition.

I have enjoyed the recent well-done research that has explored the helpful aspects of spirituality in the healing parameters of all types of medicine, including Psychiatry. It is being finely researched, but time proven that spiritual adjuncts can be helpful supports when used in the journey a patient takes to health.

I also don't disavow certain holistic approaches to improving a patient's symptoms. There are many things that can be used together to help people improve and become successful in their mental health goals. For instance sleep CD's can be useful instead of or in addition to medications for sleep.

It is important to take stock of the individual and the individual's needs and integrate a specific treatment plan from all of the available options. There is no one-cookie-cutter approach that should work for everyone.

I am so happy to share the "coins" with you that have proven to help and advance so many people on their journey to healthier living. You are getting to tap in to the inter sanctum of the world of psychiatric healing.

These are but a few of the "coins" from my practice and office.

Some things are better said in a therapy session and are better-imparted one to one.

Some things in the book can be utilized by reading them and some things may need to be clarified more in sessions or therapy.

Use what you like from the chapters. Share what you like with others. Share with me what you think about any or all of it.

Dialogue is of course what psychiatry is all about, perfecting and sharing and journeying and edifying.

Being better and being better people is what life should be all about.

# CHAPTER TWO

## The Shilling Consistency System

**Coin #2:**
Positive rewards get you further.

**Flip side:**
Consistency is everything.

One system that has had a lot of success in my practice is a consistent reward system for modification of behavior in children. I have parents and children just beaming with thanks when the program gets underway and is on track. I usually get comments of "I wish we had tried this sooner" and "It is amazing how easy this is."

There are only a few simple parts to it, but they must be done routinely, without fail, and consistently, for it to work. This means use this system and not this system and then other programs, also, at the same time.

Sometimes I have patients whose parents try to use this system and then also get so mad they spank or put the child in a corner, etc. The problem with this is that the child gets confused, and angry and hostile. This sets up more behavior issues than when you started! Pick one program and stick with it. In the beginning you won't be perfect, but keep at it. If you slip up and fall back into an old program just stop and immediately go back to this one. It will get easier and easier to do this consistently all the time.

When you show your child you can be in control and can be consistent they will develop respect for you. From respect comes more cooperation and better behavior. My system is all about consistency and it is best if it is done in a businesslike way. When emotion and screaming and yelling and hitting is removed from the process by both the parent and the child then the child can focus on the behavior they need to change, and not the emotions of the family.

It is helpful to remember that the parent is always role modeling the child. If you don't want them to yell or hit (spank) then you should not be doing that to solve problems. My program is a reward program that is consistent, positive in nature and businesslike. It eliminates the need for yelling or any other method, when used by itself and all the time.

## THE SYSTEM

## Children up to age 2/3:

REDIRECT, REDIRECT, REDIRECT. Until they are able to focus and track with you, try steering them towards something else in the room or distracting them, even multiple times, however many times you need, to some other toy or keys or cell phone music, etc. Do this whenever behaviors get out of hand or they want to pitch a fit or tantrum. So often I see parents get into a test of wills with someone several decades younger and it is just silly. The child only learns your frustration and your temper, not that you are smarter than them. Why push a point or insist they "mind" at every juncture? Pick a couple of times a day, only, to use "no" in a calm way to teach "no." Especially use this, of course, in matters of safety, but still do so calmly. If all a child this age hears is "no" all day, from an angry accumulation, it can be very defeating for them. The more positive your redirecting can be, the better it is for their self-esteem. It helps the child learn this technique in their brain files, to do later in life when things get difficult or frustrating. Remember, there will always be time when the child is a little older to do more of the instructing, in a layering fashion, of what needs to be corrected.

Children are what we call "concrete" until about the age of twelve. This means they go from "A" to "B" and "B" to "C" and are direct from one thing to another in their minds. At about the age of twelve they start to be able to "abstract" or extrapolate, or go from "A" to "E" without directly first needing "B," then "C," then "D" first to understand you. It is best then to keep the redirecting and discussion simple and "concrete" to younger children. You will be more successful, which is your goal (not the lecture you want to give, to make yourself feel better). The younger the child, the fewer words used in discipline and redirecting, the better. With "redirecting" often a minimum of dialogue works best, with just a visual of something else interesting. This is what will accomplish your goals.

## Children ages 3/4-5:

The Earn a Sticker Reward/One Warning System

## WHEN THE CHILDREN ACT UP OR DO NEGATIVE BEHAVIORS, TRY THIS:

At all times, carry STICKERS. It is best if you let the child pick out what THEY want in the way of stickers. The more special the stickers are to the child the easier this will be for you.

SHOW them the stickers for the visual connect.

Say, "This is your ONE WARNING, you need to stop this behavior now to EARN a sticker."

## Use ONLY THESE WORDS:
## ONE WARNING and EARN.

You can choose to tell them you are going to count to three or five to allow them the time to find that control mechanism within them to change their behavior. After all, your objective is to help them do so at this age. You want them to succeed. You want them to be proud of themselves for improving and finding a way to change a socially unacceptable behavior. You want them to start this process now, at this age, so they can have it all their life for success.

Give only ONE WARNING and only ONE

WARNING (do not give them a wishy-washy second and third as it makes them disrespect and have anger towards you, and only confuses them). If after ONE WARNING they do not change the behavior you simply say in a businesslike manner, "O.K., you didn't EARN a sticker," and move on. Resist doing some other punishment. You will really want to sometimes, but remember that the consistency here is the key. It really is enough that they did not EARN their reward although it may seem like not enough punishment. If you are consistent and businesslike, this system builds in its effect.

It is also important that you resist using any other word or phrasing other than the positive approach of EARN. In other words, don't say things like, "Okay now you don't get your sticker," or, "now I'm taking your sticker away," or, "now you've lost your sticker," etc. This only consternates and provokes the child, worsening the behavior. You become the "giver of good things" and they are EARNING from you, or not. Now the responsibility of it all falls all on them. This is the ultimate consequence, with either a good or bad outcome (EARN or not EARN). When you are taking things away while using other systems, or emphasizing this technique, it only makes them hate you or the action, and they don't look to themselves and their behaviors. Instead they become preoccupied with their anger towards you, the situation, or anything but focusing on what you want them to focus on, which is that of changing their behavior.

When they change their behavior after ONE WARNING, then let the CHILD peel off the sticker as part of the reward and place it on themselves or wherever they like (within reason). Later on, it is also extra reinforcing to put the stickers on a sheet of paper. This way they can always look back at the paper for reinforcement. It is good to remember that children of this age do not have a sense of time and memory in the same way as you do. This paper can be in their room where they can see it lying in bed or on the refrigerator, etc. At the end of the day you can corral the stickers as much as possible (don't be too picky about it being all of them) and make a special positive reinforcement statement of "good job" or "look how many stickers you have EARNED today for minding me." Refrain from any negative comments about how they could have done better or earned more. The reason for this is that you are trying to build self-esteem with the positive approach. The better the child's self-esteem, that they can be good, that they can change a behavior, that they can improve, the easier your job will be. The child will listen to you better and will respect you more as they have found a positive place within themselves to do so.

Some of the children in this age group will be able to do the ONE WARNING, for changing their behaviors, with the promise of a sticker, JUST at noon. Start over at noon (sticker EARNED OR NOT EARNED) with the ONE WARNING system to turn around behaviors with an EARNED sticker at bedtime. It is best to move towards this as soon as their age allows. Don't rush to it though and gage when they are able to do so.

When there are multiple children in the home they should all be on the same system for their age groups. This is even if only one child is the behavior problem. When the behavior problem child sees the other children EARNING stickers they will also want to. Do not, however, compare the children or make comments about how much better one is than the other at EARNING stickers. The children will be able to see this for themselves. Sometimes what you don't say is more important than what you do say.

## Children ages 6/7-12:

Do the ONE WARNING system. This means you give them ONLY one warning, and be sure to use the word WARNING to stop their behavior. If they stop their behavior then they are on track to EARN at the end of the designated time of EACH DAY a REWARD. This reward could be anything THEY WANT. It is best to ask them. This can be anything depending on what you can afford or have a belief system in. It can be a portion of an allowance, even a penny or a nickel they put in a jar. It can be special time with you for fifteen minutes just talking or playing, etc. To motivate them, it may need to be something they are already doing that they enjoy. If they currently are getting to watch TV or use the computer, then they need to EARN this time for these activities by stopping their negative behaviors by only ONE WARNING.

Do not keep shifting or changing the reward at whim, yours or theirs. This confusion is INCONSISTENT and just causes anger and disrespect for you in the child and your goals will not be accomplished. Try to have the REWARD be the same thing for as long as possible. As the child ages you may need to adjust the reward. At first, however, you can be sure that the child will say to you, "I don't care about earning the TV," etc. You, then, just say, "O.K. then you don't get TV." It will be interesting to see how many days it takes before they decide that maybe they do want to see some TV. Be patient and CONSISTENT on this and it will work. When they haven't EARNED their fun activity they need to go to their room where they can contemplate. As much as possible, they should not be allowed to substitute other fun things there, such as listening to music, etc. If you find the item they are to EARN is not sufficient to motivate a change of behavior, then find out what they really want and substitute it. It is best not to use food as a reward whenever possible. Sometimes this can't be avoided. When this is the case, try things like individual cheerios in a baggie or whole grain cereal pieces that they like and choose. You just don't want to start a file in their head about food as the go-to thing for rewards. This is especially true now that we are so aware of the issues with childhood obesity.

It may be that they said they wanted to EARN the TV at night but they really want computer time. They can also be given their choice of electronics, TV or computer or both, as usual, as long as the behaviors were changed with only ONE WARNING. It is important to emphasize here that you don't deviate from the words ONE WARNING. Most parents try using their own words but the kids have tuned them all out and if the words change around a lot it is not clear and CONSISTENT.

Before you start any of these systems at any age group sit down with the children and in simple terms explain to them that you are starting a new system and what its parts are.

## Children 13-30

Do the reward system in whatever creative way works. The components are for them to EARN a REWARD on a 24-hour basis for turning around negative behaviors.

It is best for REWARD time to be on a 24-hour basis and the reward to be granted CONSISTENTLY and at about the same time every day. It is important that this system not be a punishment for the parents. The parents are to pick a time of day that will be convenient for the them so it can be a consistent time. For example, with a busy hectic schedule choose a mealtime or bed time that would be fairly regular every day to do the REWARD.

An important note is that it is always best to do family discussions after a meal. It is known that 75% of all family arguments are before a meal. This is usually because everyone's blood sugar is low and people are hungry and grumpy then. It is better to eat first, then do the discussion and REWARD, or not, as they have EARNED it, or not, as the child will be more receptive. Once again, for the best results, be sure to keep the transaction businesslike.

Refrain from promising an allowance if you know you will be short on cash. The worst thing you can do with this system is promise a REWARD and not grant it for any reason. A child at any age does not get the IOU thing even though they may act like it to please you.

Be sure to pick a REWARD that YOU the parent can stick with and that doesn't require a lot of materials or inconvenience. The stickers are good for the toddlers. Be sure you are always supplied, though. Plan ahead and always have them on hand. It will be your responsibility if behaviors fall apart because the CONSISTENT REWARD is not available for the child to keep on a roll with the learning process. With the older kids something they already like doing or getting is usually the best for the REWARD. It can be, as mentioned, certain TV time each night or computer time or a choice of electronics each night as they have become accustomed to.

I would stay away from having children up to the age of twelve earn points towards something they can get later, even their allowance money, though, as it is harder for them to get the concept of delaying gratification when behavior change needs to be done. They may act like they are happy to get the nickel or dime or dollar, as you can afford, but they really don't get the immediate effect of either EARNING, or not, something immediately gratifying like their electronics. Continue their allowance if you have started one as a separate thing.

Earning cell phone or music listening device use per 24-hour period, for appropriate behavior, are a really good REWARD for teenagers. They can keep the cell phone at a designated time each day if behaviors have been appropriate, with only ONE WARNING, prior to that time, for the next 24-hours. If they have NOT earned the cell phone then they turn it over to you at the designated time for 24-hours. I can almost guarantee that a few days, now and then, without the cell phone or even the imagination of it, will produce more cooperation in appropriate behaviors, with ONE WARNING than you have ever seen before. This can also be seen with car privileges, etc. Each teenager will be different as to what they will want to EARN and it is a good idea to ask them. You want to work WITH THEM. If however the behaviors don't change with the REWARD picked then revisit what YOU think they might really want to be motivated to work for.

Sometimes it is necessary to do a contract with your child if the behaviors are so out of control or they do not grasp the concept of the system. Just get out a piece of paper. Write your child's name at the top and put the word "contract" after that. For example, write "Bobby's Contract." Then list by number the behaviors that have to change. This could be things such as:

1. Room cleaned by bedtime

2. No talking back to adults

3. No bad language or swear words

4. No arguing with brothers or sisters

5. Homework done before dinner

6. Assignments turned in at school each day

7. Curfew at 10 PM

8. Chores done as assigned

9. No yelling

10. On time for the bus or car for school

Realistically, they can get one warning for all but #6 and #7. These are what are called CONTRACT AUTOMATICS. This means it is a given that you cannot be at school to give the warning and finding out later is too late, regarding the daily turning in of assignments. It is also a given that you really can't warn about a curfew in a 24-hour period. They are either home or not. If they don't do #6 or #7, then that goes against EARNING the REWARD, AUTOMATICALLY.

It is best with a contract to set up a percentage of the items that need to be EARNED. If you have ten things, then they have to EARN 90% or nine of the items each day to get their REWARD at the designated time. This is even with the AUTOMATICS.

If any of the other behaviors become extremely repetitious, in the ONE WARNING department, then you have a discussion with the child that it is always possible to make that item an AUTOMATIC. If you need to make it an AUTOMATIC then you both need to sit down, parent and child, and amend the contract.

Anything that needs to go on the contract that is a safety issue is an AUTOMATIC. This would be things like no hitting, no destruction of property, no running away, any life threatening behavior, etc. These things would not get a warning and would result in AUTOMATICALLY not earning the

REWARD that day.

Each contract needs to be signed by each parent and each child.

It is best to have each child in the house have a contract if you go to the contract system. It won't hurt a well-behaved child to have a contract. They will just always EARN their REWARD. Also, this can be an instigation for the more behaviorally challenged child to try harder to EARN their REWARD. Be sure, though, to never compare the children verbally. Let the REWARDS do the talking. Be sure to be CONSISTENT with each child. Even the well-behaved children may have their days when they don't EARN their REWARDS. Being fair is being CONSISTENT. Gaining your child's respect will go a long way towards changing the behavior problems and the chaos in the house.

Be sure to start fresh with the CONTRACT SYSTEM and the REWARD SYSTEM.

Understandably, anger may set in with the behaviorally challenged child. Since you are the adult you should be in the position to go through whatever steps, forgiveness, etc. are needed to put the past behind you and start this with fresh eyes and a businesslike attitude.

Kids will react to YOUR ATTITUDE before they do anything else. When you are in control and when you can sit down and discuss that there will now be a contract, ask for their input (especially ask them what items need to be on the contract, as you will be surprised at what they say). Sign it and put copies up where all can recheck it, because they too will want to start fresh. You can be sure they may act like they don't want to start fresh or they may refuse to sign it or say "this isn't going to work," but just plug along with it. That is back talk; it should be on the contract, they get one warning to not say it again, today. If their attitude doesn't change it can be item #11 (good attitude). They can get ONE WARNING for attitude change also, etc. If they don't get 90% that day of what they were supposed to do on the contract, then no electronics or cell phone or whatever you decided and do it.

Be careful not to be the parent that undermines or sabotages the system.

All of the parents and stepparents need to be on the same system for it to work the best. Sometimes there is a parent who wants to be the friend and not the parent. Or this parent wants to be "the hero" parent to the child. The lack of insight in this parent can undo everything the other parents are doing. If the child thinks they can get out of the CONSISTENCY with even one parent, then they won't learn the important things from this system and it won't work.

Whenever I hear that the system isn't working, a careful review shows that one parent went rogue and is doing their own program, fell back to an old program or is trying to "improve" on this system and is adding confusing layers and extra incentives and REWARDS instead of keeping it simple.

Opponents to the system may call it "bribery" or the like. What is important to understand is that bribery is getting something in exchange for doing something illegal. This is not bribery. This is about rewards. This is about the real world. People work real world jobs to earn a reward. It is how our society is set up.

It is important for kids to understand that in our society good work earns good rewards. When you do well at work you get raises or promotions or recognition, very similar to this system. Being positive and working with and for your authority (parents, teachers, bosses, etc.) in a businesslike way gets your goals accomplished in the real world. This system is a good training ground for that.

Some children will be so biochemically ill with their condition that they cannot cooperate with the WARNING SYSTEM or the CONTRACT SYSTEM to start. These children will be those who have Bipolar Disorder or Manic Depression, Schizophrenia, Major Depression, Obsessive Compulsive Disorder, etc. They will need to see a Psychiatrist and be placed on the appropriate medications and stabilized on these medications before you can start the SYSTEMS.

You will need to start the SYSTEMS though, as soon as they are stabilized to change the behavior problems. Particularly with these children, the behavior problems have been a way of coping with a world that made sense to them, without benefit of the proper neurochemicals. They were able to manage their surroundings with their behaviors while sick. They need to find out that they will be more successful and socially acceptable with changed behaviors, when they are REWARDED for their new behaviors. It will take CONSISTENT time for this to become the new norm for them.

Don't give up. Keep at it. If you make a mistake, just get back at it. You are role modeling that you just keep trying and that is what you want them to do. It is all about CONSISTENCY.

# SAMPLE REWARD CONTRACT

1. Clean room by 8 P.M.

2. Good attitude.

3. No bad language.

4. No back talk.

5. Turn in homework daily.

6. Get along with sibs.

7. To bus on time.

8. Homework done by 8 P.M.

9. Chores as assigned.

10. Bedtime at 10 P.M.

May have one warning (not for #5, #7)

and still get reward if 9/10 (90%) are done in the 24-hours prior to 8 P.M. Can then earn electronics until bedtime. Parent to check online or by teacher note each day on homework turned in or if homework not turned in automatic loss of electronics for the designated 24-hour period.

Signatures_____

# CHAPTER THREE

## Medications

---

### Coin #3:
Take your medications daily.

### Flip side:
Chain your pill bottle/pillbox.

### Coin #4:
Keep a list of your meds on you.

### Flip side:
Include a "legend" of your pills.

Psychiatrists are doctors who go to medical school, then take four years after that to train just in Psychiatry. The additional four years in Psychiatry training is called a Psychiatric Residency. Some Psychiatrists go on for more years of specialized residency training. When a residency is completed then the psychiatrist is eligible for Board Certification. This takes approximately two more years to complete.

Because Psychiatrists are trained in this manner they can prescribe medications. This differentiates them from other mental health practitioners who do therapy but who cannot prescribe medications. For instance, Psychologists or PhD therapists provide therapy and testing but do not prescribe medications; LMHP's (Licensed Mental Health Practitioners) and MSW's (Masters in Social Work) provide therapy and testing but do not prescribe medications.

In this chapter I will address medication and medication issues. The "coins" pertaining to this chapter reflect a psychiatric practice experienced in treating many people, approximately three decades, with many types of medications, for the many diagnoses seen in a general psychiatric private practice office.

The most important thing to know about psychiatric medication is that it works best when taken regularly. This means it should be taken as prescribed and in most cases, on a daily basis.

The worst thing someone can do is to take their medication "once in a while" or "hit or miss." When you don't feel well you need to make that special effort to take your medications to get better.

I think the disconnect here for most patients is that they are familiar with things like aspirin or cold medications before they ever get prescribed a PSYCHIATRIC medication. With an over the counter cold medication or aspirin you can take it now or then. There are usually no consequences for this approach and you feel better.

However, with PSYCHIATRIC medications it is usually ineffective to take them the same way you are used to taking other things. In other words they are likely not to work if taken occasionally. Psychiatric medications are very different in that they are made to build up in your system upon regular daily use, for their best results.

Sometimes, when you miss or skip a dose of a psychiatric medication your system is thrown off. Many times when you restart your medication your system has to reprogram, so to speak, even though it has only been a day or two off of them. This can cause you to have a set back in your original symptoms, even though it might not seem obvious right at first. Patients may comment that they forgot their medications for a day and "felt fine." However, they usually report that the rest of the week was rocky and problematic. I usually have to explain to them that even though there wasn't a dramatic upheaval of symptoms from the missed dose, the effect from this type of medication can be felt days later, even though they got back on it.

It seems that medications that affect the nervous system take about thirty days for proper effect. We see this with thyroid medications, neurological medications, and psychiatric medications. Since it takes thirty CONTINUOUS days to get the proper effect to take place, even one day off throws the whole process off kilter and some restarting now has to take place again.

Another important aspect of missing psychiatric medications, for even one day, is that it can be dangerous.

Psychiatric medications are often titrated to the optimum dosage. This means that they are started at a low dose and adjusted up until the best results (alleviation of symptoms) is achieved, but at the lowest dose possible. Sometimes the lowest dose possible is a fairly high dose to help the symptoms.

When a patient forgets a dose or stops a medication suddenly, on their own, their body is ripped of something it is used to. This can cause severe symptoms and even potentially death. Some medications are habit forming or addicting. In general I search for alternatives to these types of medications. Upon occasion, patients are on these medications. When these medications are stopped suddenly the patients can experience withdrawal symptoms. Withdrawal symptoms are different and unique to habit forming or addicting medications and should not be confused with what is experienced when a patient suddenly misses other forms of psychiatric medications as I discussed above.

## SET UP A WAY TO REMEMBER YOUR MEDICATIONS!

There are many simple ways to ensure you get your medications, on time, and regularly, without missing any. This is called compliance. Look at your specific life style. If it is easier to remember your meds at night talk this over with your doctor, and if he or she agrees, take them at night. This would be the same situation if it were easier to remember them in the morning. Remembering your meds and getting them may be more important than when they were supposed to be taken, if there is any wiggle room in when to take them.

- I give people a rubber band. I suggest that they rubber band their pill bottle to something else they do routinely without fail. An example would be if you take your medications in the morning and you always brush or comb your hair at that time, then rubber band the medication bottle to the brush or comb. This would be the same at night for the toothbrush. This is called "CHAINING" your meds to something you never forget every day.

- Newer phones often have reminder bells or voices you can set for certain times of the day. Set your phone to ring you or bell you when it is time for your medications.

- Have a reliable family member help you remember to take your medications. If you do not have a phone reminder they may have one. If they do not live with you they can call you to remind you when it is medication time. Sometimes this is only necessary in the beginning until your medications help your symptoms to the point where you can eventually take over the responsibility of chaining with a rubber band or being otherwise compliant.

- Speaking of responsibility, I do not believe children or adolescents should be left to take psychiatric medications "to make them responsible." By definition they are in an age category where they need parental supervision of important things. To minimize the extra work to parents involved with this, however, it is often possible to set it up to where the kids bring (depending on age and maturity and safety issues) the medication in front of the parent, wherever they are in the house, at medication time, and show to the parent they are taking it.

- Pillboxes are a wonderful invention. When people are on multiple medications, or even on one medication they need to take more than once a day, they should put them in a pillbox. It is preferable to have the appropriate pillbox with the right compartments. This means have one that has all seven days of the week and morning, noon and night compartments. Have one day a week that you fill it from your bottles. With this system you never have a moment of wondering, "Did I take my morning pills?" "Did I take my pills tonight?" You can go to your box and check. Any busy person today can forget a medication they have to take more than once a day. All the research shows this. This is why all the pharmaceutical companies are expensively trying to make medications people only take once a day. Use your pillbox.

- When you see you only have a few pills left in your pill bottle call the pharmacy and have them call or fax your doctor for more medications or go get your refill if your pill bottle says you have more. Don't wait until you are out of medications to scramble to get more medications. It is your responsibility to keep your prescriptions current. Some offices will not fill your medications if there is a coverage doctor who does not know you when you are out.

- For little or no cost, some pharmacies will put your medications in what is called a Mediset. This is a blister pack similar to a pillbox and all you need to do is punch out your meds at the times you need them. You can always check then to see if you have taken your meds if you are not sure with a Mediset.

- Keep a list of your medications on you at all times, such as in a wallet or a purse. If you put them in your cell phone still keep a written list on your person. If there is ever an accident, someone may not be able to access the phone list. In times of emergency it is important to have a list of exactly what you are taking easily accessible. It could be life saving in an emergency room or an ambulance, when other medication choices may need to be made, drug interactions known, side effects evaluated and no other history is available.

- If you put your pills in a pillbox or Mediset, draw the pills on a piece of paper, state the color, or better yet color them, list the numbers or markings on each pill with that pill, state the name of the pill after the drawing and what it is for. Be sure to write down the dosage of your medication and how often you are to take it each day. Keep this "legend" of pills with your medications. Over time it is easy to forget which pill is for what. If you become ill for any reason someone can quickly look at this paper and understand what is in your pillbox and what you have and have not taken. Tape your legend on top of your pillbox. You can also take a picture of your pills with your phone camera and print it out and use it as your legend.

- If you ever need to go to the hospital you can easily take your pillbox/Mediset and paper "legend" with you and the time saving of it may be life saving for you. It can also help family members if they ever need to assist you if you have the flu, etc. Sometimes family members need to call the doctor for you and then they can easily identify what you are taking.

- Having a list of medications and a "legend" of what they look like can be time saving for you and your doctor when you go to various doctors just for office visits. Instead of having to list the medications on the forms at the doctor's office they will usually gladly copy your list.

- Keep your list current and accurate.

- Always tell each doctor whenever you change any medication from any doctor's office. Make your Psychiatrist aware of any new medications or of any medications you have been taken off from any other doctor's office.

Another tip that can be life saving is always open the stapled sack the pharmacist gives you at the counter or the drive through, BEFORE you leave the counter. Even if there is a line behind you, let them wait. This is so you can check to see that you got exactly the same looking pills, the same color pills, you received the last time, and the right number of pills, etc. If you are on a brand name of a medication sometimes a pharmacy can mix up and give you a generic. Many times the generic will not act the same way in your body. It will not be BIOEQUIVALENT and that is why your doctor wants you to have the brand name. The generic will look different and the name on the bottle will be different. It will say the generic name. Always tell your doctor if you get a generic and before you usually received a brand name. Better yet, have the pharmacist, then and there, before you leave, make sure it is what you are supposed to get. Many people mistakenly believe that generics are just cheaper versions for brand name medications. This is not always true with every medication. If you leave before opening your sack you will likely not be able to get an exchange for what you were supposed to get, without another charge. You can, upon occasion, get the completely wrong medication meant for someone else. So, open your sack and check.

Also, sometimes, the pharmacy doesn't have the total number of pills ordered. Read on your bottle to see if they gave you a "PARTIAL

FILL" or some of your monthly medications. If this is the case, you may need to go back to get the rest or better yet, the pharmacy can deliver to you what they didn't have, so you don't have to make another trip. It is important to know if you got your full bottle of medications as this can be confusing to you later when you are short of pills and don't know why and that you don't have to pay more to get what was just a partial filling of the original prescription.

# SAMPLE MEDICATION LEGEND

NAME, ADDRESS, PHONE NUMBER

EMERGENCY CONTACT NUMBERS/NAMES

ILLNESSES BEING TREATED:

LAST UPDATED ON_____

PRESCRIBING DOCTORS AND PHONE NUMBERS:

Medication 1___color, markings, DRAW PILL

Medication 2___color, markings, DRAW PILL

Medication 3___color, markings, DRAW PILL

Medication 4___color, markings, DRAW PILL

# CHAPTER FOUR

## Caffeine, Alcohol, Pot, Etc.

---

### Coin #5:
Caffeine is a drug.

### Flip side:
Caffeine can cause higher medication dosages.

### Coin #6:
Alcohol is liquid depression.

### Flip side:
Mixing alcohol and medications is dangerous

### Coin #7:
Pot is a sneaky self-medication.

### Flip side:
Pot can cause higher medication dosage.

Many patients tell me I am the first doctor that has asked about their caffeine usage. They then usually tell me I am the first doctor that has indicated that caffeine can interfere with the optimum work of their medications, resulting in the need for higher dosages to get symptoms under control. When you think about it, this is just common sense. Caffeine is considered a drug. It is a stimulant. It causes all of your cells to do double time, turning over and over, without breaks or rest. Your psychiatric condition is often due to a biochemical imbalance. How can making already imbalanced biochemicals, more over worked, be good for them? It is not. One way to describe it is an analogy. If your car is limping along and needs repairs you wouldn't think of gunning it up and never stopping to rest it or it might overheat, break down, fall apart, etc.

Most patients who go off caffeine completely are very pleasantly surprised. They usually were very reluctant to stop caffeine. Once they did, after a week or two, they were almost shocked at how much better they felt, how much MORE energy they had, and how much more efficient their medications were. Some patients were even able to decrease their medications.

Caffeine amounts should be reduced gradually if you have been consuming a lot of it. If you drink a cup or two a day, you may be fine just stopping it. Many people do not know which products contain caffeine or how much they actually have been getting. Caffeine is in most dark colored colas, some root beers, many green sodas and other fountain drinks, ice tea, hot tea and chocolate. You can check the labels or go on line to see if the products you have been using have caffeine. Most of the things you have been drinking come in a decaffeinated form in stores.

You can always ask for the decaffeinated
version of your favorite coffeehouse coffees.
Just say decaf before whatever you used
to order. Most teas come in decaffeinated
versions or you can order herbal teas, which
are decaffeinated. Substituting healthier
waters or juices for your sodas, now and
then, is always a good thing. One of my
patients quit her fountain drink habit and
lost seventy pounds in about a year. She
didn't change much of anything else in
her eating habits. A good way to decrease
your coffee caffeine gradually is to buy the
decaffeinated version of it and start mixing it
half and half with your regular. You can then
go with three-fourths decaffeinated coffee
then one-fourth caffeine coffee, then to all
decaffeinated. Most decaffeinated coffee
is decaffeinated by a process whereby you
can't tell the difference if it has caffeine or
not, by taste, so what's the difference. It just
takes getting used to not having that "jolt"
from the caffeine. As discussed, above, it is

better for your cells anyway. You wouldn't stick your finger in an electrical socket to get a jolt if it wasn't good for you. That little lift you get from caffeine, initially, isn't worth what it is doing to you and your medication requirements the rest of the day. So often when people feel bad they look to the immediate and not the big picture or the long term. Your recovery takes a commitment to more than just the immediate feeling a little caffeine can give you.

Often I hear patients say they just can't get going in the morning without their caffeine. This is the time to evaluate the amount of sleep you are getting. To start, your medications are likely not working efficiently due to the caffeine. Then, recognize that caffeine is well known for affecting sleep and not allowing people to sleep. It doesn't make sense, then, to be taking caffeine to wake up from not getting sleep due to caffeine! A comment I get sometimes from patients is that they stop caffeine midday or early day so it shouldn't affect them. Metabolically, as we age, caffeine affects us more than when younger. Less caffeine, and even in the early part of the day, can affect sleep (and then of course it affects the cellular imbalance anyway). Old or young, the time of day caffeine is taken is irrelevant to how it affects sleep. Caffeine is not good for sick cells trying to make a comeback with psychiatric medications no matter what time of day it is drunk.

When one eliminates caffeine via coffee, tea and soda, then sometimes a little chocolate isn't a big deal. But the operative words are "a little."

Alcohol is worthy of a book all by itself. Alcohol is classified as a "depressant." Therefore it makes no sense to pour in even a little depression when you are trying to recover as a psychiatric patient. The chemical formula for alcohol, like caffeine, can monkey with your cells so much that your medications are hard pressed to work right, often need to be increased, and multiple medications often come into play to deal with it. How can drinking alcohol be worth all of that when the objective to get better is so easily derailed by a drink?

Some psychiatric conditions are hallmarked by people self-medicating with alcohol. They find a quick fix with how they feel after a drink. However, they don't associate how bad they feel later with the residual effects of the alcohol as it continues to metabolize and then wreak havoc on their system hours and even days later. This discussion is even about a single drink. Let's extrapolate that to those who really over imbibe with many drinks.

So often I hear about people being proud of keeping this self-medicating to certain days or not when they work, etc. What gets missed is that subsequent days after drinking, there is still a hangover, and it is the hangover's effects that patients are in denial about. These hangover days are just as damaging to the body and to the mind and to patient lives in general.

It is really helpful to give your Psychiatrist an alcohol free period in which to start a medication so as to titrate it or to see how it affects your system alone. It makes it nearly impossible to tell what is the lowest dose of medication you need and when to adjust to the next dosage if alcohol and other substances are at play in your system.

It seems that with certain conditions and the types of medications used for them, that even a single drink of alcohol cancels out the effects of the medications. Patients sometimes compound this by deciding not to take their medications when they drink. Then they are really set up for a decline in their condition. It is best not to use alcohol when on psychiatric medications. I suggest people order Perrier (a brand of fizzy water), with a lime, one of the non-alcoholic beers such as those made by O'Douls, Beck's, Budweiser's, or Coor's, etc. a longneck root beer, cranberry juice in a wine glass, water with a twist of lemon, decaffeinated cola, or any mixed drink without the alcohol (virgin pina colada, etc).

It has long been known that mixing alcohol with psychiatric medications is dangerous anyway. This is due usually to what is called potentiation. Potentiation means that alcohol or the medication can make one or the other more powerful. You may not be able to gage the powerfulness of the combination: you could stop breathing, have an irregular heartbeat and you could die. One need only look to recent news stories of several celebrities to know how true this is.

If you cannot take a break from alcohol to start a medication, have found that you have struggled with alcohol in the past or in general you think your use of alcohol has affected your daily life, a good recommendation is to seek a networking group that deals with this. The research shows that AA has the best track record. It is free. It is in the phone book in your area under Alcoholics Anonymous. There are many, many meetings and many meeting types from which to choose. You do not have to think you are an alcoholic to attend. If alcohol has been affecting your life, get help from the experts who deal with it. AA is a good adjunct to your work with your Psychiatrist. It helps you to get off to a good start if you need medications and have trouble starting them off alcohol. If you have had a bad experience with a treatment program or an AA meeting in the past, try a different kind. There are so many different forms of meetings that there is one that will fit your needs. If you find you need an inpatient treatment program that is also an option. Another alternative that has worked for a lot of people and is less costly is doing ninety AA meetings in ninety days. When inpatient treatment is not possible, this has been a remarkable substitute for many, if the factors are right.

Pot is similar in its problems for the psychiatric patient. Much has been written lately in the research about how it negatively affects the biochemicals the psychiatric medications are so valiantly trying to help. What is unique to pot is that it remains in drug screens for two weeks and thus in the system of the individuals. One hit of pot and it is two weeks of trying to deal the best with the psychiatric symptoms by psychiatric medications now at a handicap for weeks. Pot is another sneaky self- medication. It initially makes people think they feel better. It then slowly continues to mess with the cells and what they are able to do for weeks, when they need to only be receptive to the proper medications that can really help. AA continues to be a good reference and recommendation to patients to help with those who find pot, or any other drug, adversely affecting their lives.

I view caffeine, alcohol and pot to mere band-aids for a condition that needs the surgery of real psychiatric medications.

These substances only make for walking wounded. Visualize the walking wounded, band-aided by alcohol, pot and caffeine, when they could have had the proper surgery for their conditions, and gone on to a better life.

# CHAPTER FIVE

## Be the Barracuda

---

### Coin #8:
The barracuda is not what you think.

### Flip side:
Assertiveness is good.

I tell my patients that there are three types of fish in the sea:

1. There are the passive tiny schools of fish that skitter off when you get in the water.

2. There are the aggressive predatory sharks.

3. Then there is the barracuda.

The barracuda has gotten a bad rap. It is not in the same category as the aggressive shark. The barracuda hangs out in its own space, takes care of it's own self and protects itself only if it's space is invaded. The barracuda holds on to it's own area, it has established its boundaries and feels entitled to have and to manage it's own area. In a sense you could say the barracuda is a metaphor for self-esteem or self worth.

Regardless, my point here is to discuss when people get in to passive aggressive situations in life and go to extremes when there is a middle ground. They are either too passive or too aggressive. These extremes usually don't serve them well. The extremes often get them in trouble or don't advance what they want their goals to be. When people get a sense of "being the barracuda" they develop a way of owning their space and their self. Then their goals naturally advance. They are less likely to succumb passively to situations. They are less likely to succumb to the people that buffeted them before and got them off their game. When people focus on being the barracuda they also don't go aggressively into things that then usually backfire on them, due to the excessiveness of the approach. Having a strong sense of your self in an assertive way, or as the barracuda, always puts you in a good position to state your case or defend your territory, in a businesslike way. Being the barracuda allows you to feel entitled to exist with your opinions on something and persevere. It takes practice to "become the barracuda" when you have grown up socialized to be passive or aggressive, or a combination of both. This is when it helps to have a phrase like "be the barracuda" at the ready in your mind. When you want to fall back on old ways, pull out the phrase, and say to yourself "BE THE BARRACUDA." This will help you right yourself quickly and hold your own ground again, in the healthier way.

Women sometimes have been socialized to grow up rather passively. It helps them to recognize this and move towards being more assertive, like the barracuda. It takes practice to change a habit. Some research shows it takes two weeks of constant endeavor to change a habit.

The down side to being passive is that an abundance of being passive can sometimes lead to a sudden episode of aggressiveness.

The people around you get confused and a lack of communication ensues, arguments commence and original goals do not get accomplished. Passive/Aggressive communication tends to get into the non-verbal communication styles. This can be body language or pay back styles. It is always better to be direct and businesslike and verbal. Don't count on anyone "getting" your non -verbal hints or cues. Usually, it only leads to misunderstandings. Passive/ Aggression also tends to get into gamey game playing that seems to have no end. This can be seen in the work place or in families.

It is always best for everyone to be direct, businesslike and communicate assertively. It cuts down on the usual misunderstandings otherwise seen.

Always keep things resolved in an assertive businesslike way. If you think someone is trying to communicate with you in a Passive/

Aggressive way, ask him or her to talk about what is bothering them. Ask them if there is something the two of you should discuss and resolve. Don't let things fester or participate in the Passive/Aggressive games.

Those who tend towards the aggressive often are really being bullies. They think their best defense is an offense. They usually are paranoids who think they need to get the jump before someone else does. They will always eventually be found out for what they are, so it is best for them also to move towards the more assertive approach.

Those in families and the work place who are dealing with the passive and the sneaky or overtly aggressive bullies are aware of their tactics. As you persevere, being the persistent barracuda, in a positive way, will always serve you best.

The next chapter will give you even more

tips on how to be the best at being assertive to accomplish your goals.

# CHAPTER SIX

## Assertiveness Training

Coin #9:
Use the word "I" when being assertive.

**Flip side:**
The focus of assertiveness is to change you.

When first learning to be more assertive start sentences with the words:

> "I feel,"

or > "I think,"

OR THE BEST IS: "I would be happy if."

Examples of this would be, "I feel hurt when you yell at me." The other party may be ready with a come back but you need to remain assertive and calm and businesslike and respond again with an identification of how their response makes you feel. What is important about this is that you are establishing your territory as being valid. You are establishing your feelings as being valid. You are helping them see you as another person with feelings and validity and opinions that count. You are not engaging in aggressive arguing back but are moving the conversation towards assertive resolution.

The first few times you do this with someone

who is aggressive or who is used to being loud and argumentative with you, they may just leave in a huff. They do not know how to handle the new assertive you. Be sure, however, they will be thinking about how you did not become passive or that you did not aggressively argue back. They will be mulling over the mature control you now show. The healthier they are the more likely they will not try their old tactics quite so much any more. They now know you have new tools. They may test you again. Just don't engage. Stay assertive. State your feelings and thoughts. Stay businesslike.

The most unhealthy opponents may ramp up their aggression. Stay assertive. Do whatever is healthy on your part and stay assertive.

Assertiveness is about being direct, open, and honest. It is about being socially appropriate. It is about standing up for your rights; all while you are respecting the rights of others.

Key words and phrases are important to assertiveness.

When you express your feelings verbally, you have started the dialogue of assertiveness. Many people are not in touch with their feelings. They need to do work first on identifying their feelings. They need to feel it is fine to have feelings and that it is fine to express them. Some people come from families where they were not allowed to express their feelings. Some people think that if they say out loud that they are angry, they will go further than that and lose control and become very angry. Just the opposite usually happens. When you can verbalize how you feel, it mitigates or makes that emotion smaller, so you can consciously deal with it better.

I tell people to start by practicing in your car alone. When another driver makes you mad, say assertively out loud, "that makes me mad," or "that makes me angry." Get used to how it sounds. Practice it. You can say it to your young children; try saying out loud "that makes mommy angry" or "that makes mommy sad when you do that." When this is said in a businesslike tone, it is a way of teaching and will be listened to. You will be surprised at how much your children just want to know how you feel about things, that they don't know until you tell them, and how it keeps problems resolved.

Feelings that can be identified include: happy, sad, glad, mad, angry, frustrated, pleased, etc. When you are truly being assertive you will find yourself using all of these words and more.

Assertiveness training also includes using the words "I understand" to others.

You can identify to others that you understand how they feel or what they said, or what they must be going through, etc. You first use the word "I" to establish that you are in the conversation, while recognizing that they are too. You are establishing that there will be a discussion involving you and them and both of your feelings and thoughts.

Assertiveness is rounded out by being able to use the phrase "I want."

It is important when you are assertive to get your needs met. Start again with the word "I." Then plug in what it is you need to get your goals met. Examples may be "I want you to behave better," "I want time to think about this," "I need more information," etc.

When you start a phrase with "It would make me happy if," or "I would be happy if," then you are working to get your needs met. This is the best phrase to use, whenever possible, because it gives the other person the opportunity to choose it to be their idea to make you happy. It is not a phrase that sounds critical to anyone. It is not a phrase that is demanding or nagging or telling someone what to do. It seems to be phrasing that connects with people's brains, allowing them to take notice of what you are going to say next. This is step one to getting across your request. You can then more easily get your needs met.

Using the word "would" instead of "could" also helps when being assertive. Some people chafe at the word "could." It engenders, "are they able?" which sounds critical of their abilities. When you ask, "would," then you are giving them the option of doing something without the psychological unconscious/subconscious baggage of "if they are capable or not," in a critical way.

This may seem like splitting hairs on a few simple words, when the motivations behind the speaker are the same. However, research isn't done for nothing. The studies show that better, less complicated and more effective assertive communication takes place when we are aware of these few things and put them in practice.

There are many rewards to learning the assertive approach to life, and it is worth changing old habits to do so. Remember though, when you become assertive, the endpoint is not that it will change the other person but what it will be doing for you. Personally, it will be giving you a healthier, happier, more centered and grounded sense of self that has validity, and a sense of self where you are entitled to feelings that will be heard and discussed. It is interesting, though; that many times when you learn assertiveness, there is a change in others around you, too.

# CHAPTER SEVEN

## The Care and Feeding of Women

---

**Coin #10:**
Respect will get you everything.

**Flip side:**
Women's relationships are like gardens.

The previous discussions of assertiveness have mentioned women and socializations. The research has indicated that women are often heavily socialized towards the passive side and women can become more accomplished in their goals when leaning from the passive/aggressive towards the assertive. Men and other women listen better to what is being said when emotion is removed from the discussion and information is presented in the assertive format.

I will also discuss here other things that are important to know about relationships with women. These will be true with female friendships as well as with male/female relationships.

Recently, I was asked to do a TV piece on "What Women What." Easily, the first answer I gave to the interviewer, a male, was "security." He took this to mean financial security. He said something like, "So we need to have the big job right?" Actually, security means so much more. A woman can feel secure in a relationship when truth and fidelity are the hallmarks. When women are polled on this, eventually this is what comes to the forefront.

A woman's self-esteem is what usually requires a suitor to not be in a certain triad of "no job, no car, and living at home with mom." The self-esteem naturally takes care of the financial eventually, by the very nature of a woman looking for a mate who also has the self-esteem to provide for himself.

Self-esteem and the need for security usually involves a woman wanting to feel cared for, wanting to be listened to, and wanting to be placed in an appropriate priority. In other words, a woman likes to be shown respect. Women see respect as a sign of security in a relationship.

It is respectful to care about a woman's opinions or at least listen to them for discussion.

It is respectful to care about a woman's time management issues and offer to help with them or ask what would be the most helpful.

It is respectful to keep track of a woman's favorite interests, and then encourage them with notes, words, gifts, etc. For guys it is often helpful to keep a list of the hints she gives on "oh, I like this or that" in your phone or on paper. Guys do not usually keep lists in their heads as easily as women do. A woman will really take notice if someone has shown they have been thinking about her and have taken the time to foster an interest of hers. This does not have to be pricey or even involve money. Women will however, at times, be aware of financially disrespectful gifts as this can be a set back in a relationship.

I once had a woman complain to me in session that she was very hurt when she received a two-dollar wooden salad/fork set from a wealthy boyfriend for a holiday. If she had hinted she wanted that item she would have been very pleased he had listened and put it on his list to get for her. However, if such an item were not a hinted for gift for a special occasion, then it becomes disrespectful, solely from the "not knowing her interests," angle.

Women don't usually mind "frivolous gifts" that may cost a little more, even when they say don't want them. At issue here is the concept of gifting language. I use the example of a dozen roses. There really isn't any reason for them, they usually cost more than they should, they won't last, etc. They are "frivolous." However, the gift language is one of caring and respect towards the recipient. The gift language is also one of giving sacrificially by the giver.

This somehow creates a sense of security in the recipient. If someone is willing to show respect by consideration, thought, time and some sacrifice. It secures a person that they have meaning and value to someone when that someone can show they care by giving thoughtful trivial things like gifts. It follows in many women's thinking that when a suitor can show the woman has meaning and value to them by humoring them in small instances or trivial gifts, then the suitor will be able, reliable and receptive in the more important things in life as they come up. Consider the trivial accomplishments as a trial run for the woman as to the abilities of the suitor to fulfill small and important needs. Women will take in to account the financial situation of the suitor. For some a single rose or a heart shaped pizza will be a stretch financially or sacrificially, and this would mean as much.

I think this is why missing birthdays or

anniversaries is such a big deal to a lot of women. There would have been a message in the gift if she had been given one but there is even more of a message when one is not even received. It is not much of a psychological stretch to believe that a little thoughtful gift now and then goes a long way, or that forgetting to give one lends the woman to think she's being disrespected.

Since men (and some women) do not naturally keep lists of important dates or favorite interests in their heads, and since this seems to be an important thing in relationships, like it or not, keep them on your computer, in your phone with reminders, with your secretary, on a calendar, or by any means that keeps you ahead of the belated, "I'm sorry I forgot but you must know how much I care" scenario. I am saving you a lot of grief. You can never go wrong with showing kindness and consideration and respect towards anyone. You do not want to forget it towards someone you especially care about and may have come to take for granted, a little.

It holds true today, just like the women of yore, that woman like to "throw down the gauntlet" a bit.

This means they like their suitor to work a little bit for their affections. Suitors no longer have to joust in heavy armor or slay dragons to do so, but a little frivolous gift or attention might do. However, it needs to not be infrequent. So many times I hear women's concerns that they have noticed their suitor has stopped being attentive once married or have entered in to a committed relationship. Women like to throw down the gauntlet and men like to win. Since men are goal directed, once they have won the prize, they at times do not think they need to still run the gauntlet. In couples counseling I like to help the suitors understand that even though the original gauntlet accomplishes one goal, i.e., marriage, moving in together, etc., they now have a new goal. The new goal is to keep the woman happy. Yes, they still have to do the courtship things to satisfy and accomplish the new goal; that of keeping their gal happy.

This is a good place to reinforce that infidelity can create insecurity, which is the opposite of your goal. It goes without saying that security gets shattered when dishonesty is the foundation of a relationship. You can't have infidelity without dishonesty. There is no way in a double life to reassure a partner that they are your focus and give them their security. Inconsideration to a partner is integral with infidelity and creating insecurity. With all the disease out there, someone who is seeing multiple partners is risking the health of all of the partners. There is no way to be sure that "someone on the side" doesn't have Herpes or AIDS or Venereal Warts, or Trichomoniasis, or Syphilis, etc. or a combination of several of these, and other conditions. It is always helpful to bear in mind that when you have sex with someone, or kiss someone, you are kissing or having sex with everyone they have ever seen.

You don't know what their former partners may have had, if the extra person your partner is seeing has something, or if the person you have on the side has something despite appearing healthy. When you bring this silent dishonesty home to an unsuspecting partner, it is not only disrespectful, inconsiderate and dishonest, it could be deadly. This is why security and trust is so important to a woman. It is fundamental to know that the person you think cares about you, honestly does so.

Women to woman friendships are particularly complicated at times. I like to indicate to people that they are a lot like gardens. When you think of them this way it helps to eliminate some of the heartache I hear about friendship problems.

For healthy gardens you always have to add new plants. Women should plan to add new friends all the time to their "friend garden."

For healthy gardens you need to weed occasionally. If you have a "weed" or a negative toxic friend who is a bad influence or who is bringing you down, you can distance yourself or "weed" them out of your garden, to keep it healthy.

A healthy garden needs to be watered and fertilized. Your friends need to be cared for and fed - sometimes literally, sometimes figuratively. This is why women lunch. This is why women buy each other little gifts or cards. This is why women talk to each other and support each other. Efforts of caring and nurturing make friendships and gardens grow.

Healthy gardens need to be tended to. Healthy friendships need to be constantly tended to, to keep women friendships alive. Checking in and keeping in touch are important aspects of tending that are essential to the growth and well being of the wonderful entity known as the female friendship.

# CHAPTER EIGHT

## A Healthy Man

---

**Coin #11:**
Men need den time.

**Flip side:**
Healthy individual time can mean
better togetherness.

**Coin #12:**
Security (see Chapter Seven) can decrease
those pesky phone calls.

**Flip side:**
Distance doesn't always mean disinterest.

A common complaint in the office from women is that their guy doesn't always want to be with them. This causes suspiciousness, fears and insecurities.

A fundamental need of the male species is to have "cave time" or time alone, or time with other guys. There is a reason why that room in your house is called the "den." It is helpful for women to understand that their relationships will actually be stronger if both she and he develop individual self-interests that feed their souls and utilize their gifts. Some alone time for both speaks to a healthy relationship. It is usually very important for the male species to have time to cultivate their male interests. The more their gal understands this the better their relationship will usually be.

This is of course as long as the guy's "away time" doesn't involve infidelity of any type, which usually weakens the relationship.

The time spent back together can then involve mutually compatible things for the best relationships. This isn't to say both partners may need to tolerate a hobby or interest of the other. Some compromise is a given in any relationship. The saying "opposites attract" does seem to be true. Often one partner thinks the other "completes them" with their differences. This is all good as long as there is a healthy amount of compatibility in other areas.

Many times I hear from guys in treatment that they are very irritated by their gals calling them all the time and they want to know why.

This goes back to things previously discussed in the previous chapters. Women think differently than men. Women usually like to be called and connected with, listened to, and checked in with, to let them know they are being thought about. This is what they are doing with you. Since most guys don't think like this, it is confusing to them and often irritating.

A solution can be to discuss one or two calls a day. This could be a call at lunch breaks, once a day, unless an emergency requires more. Also, when there is "listening time" when you get back together, this seems to diminish the need for so many extra calls. This comes back to the security issues discussed in a previous chapter. It takes time to develop this, but it will help. Visa versa, it helps the relationship for the female to encourage the male individual time. Male individual time makes for a healthier male who is then in a better state to meet the female's needs when they get back together at couple time.

Men need friendships too. This helps foster a healthier individual. Men will likely cultivate their friendships differently than women. Having a range of buddies and activities to trade off of can be a healthy good thing, as long as there aren't any toxic, negative relationships that jeopardize the positive big picture. A sign of maturity and a healthy male is to focus on the positive individual hobbies and pursuits and the buddy relationships that edify and don't bring problems or conflicts.

# CHAPTER NINE

## Families

Coin #13:
Family support can greatly help recovery.

**Flip side:**
Family can give important history.

Coin #14:
Family therapy can help a sick family.

**Flip side:**
Motives to avoiding family therapy
should be examined.

Coin #15:
Biological parents should be the family
disciplinarians.

**Flip side:**
Stepparents should not try to take the
place of biological parents.

## Coin #16:
Children need to hear positives
about ex-spouses.

## Flip side:
Family talk should not be bullying.

## Coin #17:
AA, AL-ANON, ALATEEN can help
along with your therapy.

## Flip side:
Substitute a new family if you need to.

I have seen healthy mature supportive family units/members as being one of the biggest single aids to people recovering from any condition. This holds true for the patients recovering from mental illness.

Many times it is the family member/ significant other who brings the patient in to the appointment, sits supportively in the waiting room during the appointment or even comes in with them for a few minutes at the beginning of the appointment, if the patient allows. This can be quite valuable. Some mental health conditions, by their nature, and their biochemical makeup, make it very difficult for the patient to initiate appointments or even get to an appointment or go to places unaccompanied (they usually take someone they trust).

Family can also fill in the history for psychiatric conditions that the patient is either too ill to remember or is in denial of.

This history from a caring family member can mean everything in the way of an accurate diagnosis.

For example, many times patients who have Bipolar Disorder/Manic Depression only make it in to see the Psychiatrist when they are depressed. When this patient is in their manic phase they feel really good, usually too good, and they don't see the need for help as their judgment is quite clouded. When the patient starts to feel depressed and then seeks help they may only tell the doctor, then, that they are depressed. They leave out the part about their prior manic behaviors of spending sprees, bankruptcy, never sleeping, irritability, frequent job changes, explosive anger, etc. These things, however, are foremost in the minds and concerns of the family that brought them in. When the doctor can get the entire picture of symptoms from the family, a more accurate diagnosis can be made and then the more appropriate medication can be chosen for this condition.

If just an antidepressant is chosen for someone with Bipolar Disorder/Manic Depression, because only depression is seen and reported, then actually the manic symptoms can be made worse. Usually, this patient needs a mood stabilizer first, which is a different medication from an antidepressant.

Sometimes after a mood stabilizer is started and adjusted well, there can still be a need for an antidepressant. The mood stabilizer, however, should be there first, when possible.

Often, family can give a more accurate history when it comes to the level of substance abuse actually taking place by a patient. This can also be important as it can be life saving. Mental health patients often under-report the amount of alcohol or other drugs/

substances they may be abusing. The doctor needs to know exactly what the patient is taking and how much, so an accurate and safe treatment plan can be devised with prescriptions. As previously mentioned, the mixing of prescription medications and alcohol/drugs can be dangerous.

Certain types of depressions require that family or significant others bring patients in. This is seen in norepinephrine deplete or psychomotor retarded depressions and certain types of anxiety and panic disorders.

Psychomotor retarded depressions have nothing to do with mental retardation. It is the motor retardation or slowness of movement that is referred to here. This depression is hallmarked by an inability to get up and go and do things. Often there is excessive sleeping. The patient is so unable to motivate that they usually cannot make or get to appointments themselves. If an appointment is made they need a family member to make sure they keep it. The patient is just so tired and down and slow that they usually are not caring for themselves and someone else needs to initiate the treatment appointments and medications until their natural biochemicals are improved and can then help them make sense to do so on their own.

Those who suffer from anxiety and panic sometimes need the companion family member to feel safe to journey to unfamiliar offices and surroundings. Sometimes these patients cannot take public transportation alone due to fears, nor can they drive themselves.

Having family as part of the therapy team can be very helpful in an accountability way, also. This can be done with the individual therapy or with family therapy sessions. Certain psychiatric conditions lend themselves to patients who say they are taking their medications when they are not, or they are doing goals when they are not. When family and the patient and the doctor are all together for part or all of a session, accountability sets in. This is when everyone in a patient's environment is on the same page, and compliance is more likely for this patient's success.

Family therapy is a separate type of session where the focus is to involve the whole family for the session.

Family therapy is particularly helpful, at times, as the dynamics of the family change when there is a trained professional involved. More can be accomplished than when the families just get together on their own and fight or continue in non-productive patterns towards each other.

When consent forms are signed and family

therapy sessions are video taped, it is quite dramatic to see the changes. This change is particularly seen in the family bully. Much more can be accomplished in a shorter period of time with videotaping. When honesty prevails, that is when healing or problem solving can really take place. People also tend to listen more, instead of thinking what their next sentence will be, in family therapy. In family therapy people know on some level that there is a neutral professional and if the video is involved, there is also a witness to any patterns and manipulations. Primarily, the lies previously told and maintained get revealed and dealt with.

When family members refuse to be involved in family therapy then the motive as to why needs to be looked at.

Sometimes family therapy is court ordered/ recommended for various reasons. When the responsible parties don't set this up or certain family members are resistive to doing the therapy then there is secondary gain to the motive of the resisters. Someone is usually fearful their lies will be revealed, the truth will come out, and that they will not be able to continue to control, manipulate and bully. This may have worked so well for them, sometimes not only in just a family system but in an entire community. I was privy to one such a scenario - the results were a family's elderly parents went to their graves without ever knowing the truth about what certain family members were up to or what lies had been told them about other family. The elderly parents suffered terribly at their deaths. Initial family therapy could have staved off an avalanche of problems and heartache and suffering.

One of the most difficult family issues dealt with in a psychiatry office is that of stepchildren and stepparents.

It is usually best to have the biological parents be the disciplinarians. I suggest family meetings for all the family members when there is a biological parent and a stepparent or a "significant other" parent figure (taking a stepparent role). At this family meeting (it should always be after a meal when arguments are less likely and blood sugars are more settled) it needs to be established that both the biological parent and the other parent figure recognize that the children have two distinct BIOLOGICAL parents (and even if one is deceased).

Why this is important is that kids KNOW this. They know this even if they have never met one of their biological parents, have met and dislike one of their biological parents, or like both their biological parent and stepparent, etc. They still have some connection to their original blood parent. This is subconscious or unconscious or on whatever basis, but it is there. Consciously, a child can even say they see their stepparent as more of a parent than the absent or semi-absent biological parent. They may even say they consider their stepparent their true parent. But, underneath it all, they still believe they have two biological parents that should be responsible for them. This goes back to my chapter where I discuss in more depth the concrete nature of how children think.

So, once you have established that you have acknowledged that the child has two biological parents, the next step is to state that the biological parent in the home is going to be the main disciplinarian.

Next you state that the stepparent/significant other is there, as the other adult, only to BACK UP THE BIOLOGICAL PARENT'S DISCIPLINE PLAN.

Now you state that the stepparent/significant other is not there to replace the biological

parent but is there to be an adult FRIEND
to the child, but with the distinction that, as
the other adult, they are to follow and back
up the biological parent's discipline plan for
the home.

This is all necessary as it decreases the
resentment seen in so many blended
families by the children, about being told
what to do by non-relatives. It decreases
the hostility towards the available biological
parent and the non-biological member.
Sometimes children take out unconscious
and subconscious anger towards an "absent"
parent on the available parents. The family
meeting can establish that the family
wants to move in a positive direction, with
everyone understanding each other, as
much as possible. The family meeting can
establish that the non-family member is
not going to be in a competing role with an
already biological parent, but will be there
as a mentor/friend, and will be consistent

in discipline as BACKUP, with the biological parent.

Now it is up to the biological parent and the non-biological parent figure to put together a discipline plan or house rules they both can stick to and be consistent with. See my chapter on this. When the biological parent is not present, and it is up to the stepparent/ significant other to follow the discipline plan, it is helpful if that adult does so bearing in mind that they are the FRIEND/MENTOR. This will garner more cooperation between them and the child. The rules, rewards and consequences are all the same. It is just administered with a different mind set by all and works much better without all the underlying drama and angst and hostilities. Goals are better met by all. Relationships are better for all in a more workable family unit.

Something else that is very helpful on this subject is to be mindful of the conversation type and conversation subjects that are the most conducive to having healthy blended families.

Sometimes, it is very hard during a break up to find something positive to say about the ex-partner. It depends on the situation of the break up or the character of the other person. It is ESSENTIAL, however, for the sake of the psyche of your children to find some real, honest, positive things to say about the ex-partner in front of the children. This is a self-esteem building tool for your child and it can not come from any other source.

Your child develops a sense of self-esteem or sense of self from both BIOLOGICAL parents (no matter how great a substitute a stepparent is, this stepparent helps in mentoring but can not fill this part of it completely). Any positive thing you can say about your ex-partner for your child, to take away as a building block for his/her character, will be doing a service to that child. Even if the ex-partner parent is in prison, you can say things like "your dad was a really good artist," or "he was so caring to your grandma" or "your mom was such a good cook" or your "mom was always so punctual," etc. This does not take away from gentle discussions about right and wrong and if an ex-partner did something you don't want your child to emulate and you want them to learn from that person's mistake. Discussions of this nature should be businesslike and without as much emotion and drama and anxiety as possible. They should be instructional in nature. When a child gets older they can draw their own conclusions about the ex-partner/parent and they will. While their self-esteem is being formed, as a child, they need to know the positives about both BIOLOGICAL parents so as to become the best character from both. If all they hear is that one parent is really bad because of this or that, like a constant mantra, then it can affect deep down what that child thinks they are made of. It is better for them to have something positive to use as a building block for forming their self-image.

It is important to watch our language with each other in both blended and non-blended families. Sometimes I cringe when I watch sitcoms. So often there is this role modeling of the perfect family in a sitcom and then they are trash talking each other. They "tease," call each other names, or put each other down to get another bump from the laugh track. The problem with this type of put down and teasing is that in a real family it is a type of bullying. The words are hurtful and it does not make for a harassment free, positive environment. It is better in a family for everyone to be encouraging of each other, accentuating the positive, and trying to build each other's self-esteem and making each other the best they can be. Otherwise, the motives and emotional maturity need to be examined. It wouldn't make for a very good sitcom, but a healthy happy child, wife and husband might be preferable to a laugh track any day.

Family dynamics can become complicated when there is a scapegoat child or one family member breaks free of a sick family syndrome and becomes upwardly mobile and then unwilling to participate in the previous family dysfunction.

Some families, not necessarily consciously, choose to scapegoat or victimize a child. This is a child that the other children, and sometimes the parents, verbally and non verbally tend to pick on and put down and place blame on, to maintain the family on some sort of dysfunctional but working plane. This can also be seen in some work places with a worker. In the family system it is naturally damaging to the child and really to the other family members to persist in such a way. It is helpful to get the child a mentor, an aunt or uncle or someone outside of the family system to be a positive influence and to be a dynamic system changer and support system. When a scapegoat child breaks free of such a family system, the other family members have to juxtapose to find a new family equilibrium, where they continue to avoid responsibility for their problems or issues by scapegoating someone else or best case scenario, they start to take responsibility because their scapegoat is gone.

Today we have organizations such as AL-ANON and ALATEEN, Adult Children of Alcoholics, Big Brothers and Big Sisters, Teammates, etc., that give children and adults the opportunity to distance themselves from dysfunction in their families and gain positive mentoring or tools, from which they can learn ways to move on from a negative family system. AL-ANON, Adult Children of

Alcoholics and ALATEEN are organizations for the family and friends of alcoholics. They are wonderful organizations that help family and significant others deal with the dysfunction that alcoholic family members can bring into a family home. When the family dysfunction is alcoholism or drug abuse, or some other addiction, the non-using family member/members can be the ostracized ones, as they do not play along with that family's script. The non-using family member usually puts people first as a priority. The using family members have primarily one priority and it is a substance. It can be several substances, and/or the money in an estate or gambling or anything but people and people's feelings. It usually takes a lot of work in AA or other very long-term treatment programs for users or alcoholics to gain the honesty and insight to change. While they are working this program it is very helpful for the non-using members of the family to work with their healthy support systems available. Non-users are givers by nature and it is hard for them to understand the mindset of users since they do not come from that ilk. The givers tend to take the slights and mistreatments of user family members personally. It is helpful for the non-using family members to understand how different the mind set is of the user (and not even a family member can be a priority to someone who has a single-minded focus to get just their needs met or their fix, be it alcohol or drugs or money or high from another inanimate source). Sometimes it takes years of therapy for people to grasp this concept. They just continue to be in so much pain from the missed outings and missed birthdays and missed child support from the user parent. Or they continue to be depressed by the discounting of feelings by the user spouse or sibling. Understanding the nature of the user and their inability to put any feelings or priority into anyone else, will help the non-user family member move on to make their own healthy life, not personalize it into their self-esteem which they should not, and will help them avoid needless further pain. I know of one situation where a childless aunt invested a lot of support and mentoring into nieces and nephews and siblings. The efforts were generally met with indifference, and they left her in the lurch during a serious family matter, confusing the aunt, until the concepts thusly discussed here were understood. The aunt's generosity stopped to the user family members and she focused her energies on those who appreciated and understood giving intentions, and on those who understood people as priorities and who understood kindness as a focus. The users were oblivious, as their mindset was so elsewhere as a priority. It is healthy to accentuate the positive and distance oneself from the negative, toxic family/significant other relationships.

Becoming upwardly mobile, and suffering consequences as a result within a dysfunctional family system is somewhat unique to our day and age. Educational opportunities are more available now through a variety of sources for those who have the integrity and abilities, and we are seeing this develop as a new phenomenon.

It is only in recent years that we have seen the opportunities in certain ethic groups and genders to excel past what was the usual and customary expected of a certain family. This is called upwardly mobile.

Many times now we hear of people saying they are the first to graduate from high school or college in their family. We now see men and women of all races enter into graduate programs for the PhD and M.D. and J.D. degrees that before were not so common, except in certain family systems where many prior relatives with these degrees had gone before them.

Depending on the emotional strength and maturity of the other family members, and their individual security as to who they feel they are, the upward mobility of a family member can be viewed in two ways.

When the family is healthy and the members are secure about themselves and what they do, the upward mobility is generally met with a positive attitude and a supportive family reinforcement. If a brother is a bus driver but he is secure in being the best bus driver he knows how to be, then he is glad for his sibling when he graduates from law school as an attorney.

However, if the sibling is an insecure secretary who might not see himself as the best secretary possible he could take an evil spiteful turn and try to bring down a sibling he sees as becoming successful. I know of one situation where a sister distinguished herself by becoming a doctor, the first in her family to have a graduate degree. A sister who was a schoolteacher took it upon herself to call hospitals the doctor sister worked in with intent to cause trouble for the upwardly mobile sister. The upwardly mobile sister could not dumb down enough to make the insecure sister less insecure or less petty. She could not give up her degree to try to fit back into a family system. She had excelled past a family system that did not keep up in its maturity or emotional IQ. What is left in such circumstances is to opt for family therapy if a situation has become out of hand. If the petty party refuses to participate in family therapy then other options need to be looked at.

One option is to stay within the family system with certain healthy family members as much as possible, distancing from the unhealthy members in a hybrid fashion.

Another option is to leave a sick family system and create your own family from a "family" of your own choosing. If I am quoting Oprah Winfrey correctly, I believe she once said she decided to do this. When your own family does not or can not live up to a healthy functioning family unit, you need to create for yourself that support system out of people who have proven they make the grade. You don't necessarily need to tell people you have decided that they are now your mother or father or brother figure. But, if you have a mentor at church or a great neighbor who is like a mom or a sister to you, they can be your new family. You probably have already formed family-like ties with these people as they have proven to be healthy, supportive, caring individuals you can count on when needed. You don't have to stay within unhealthy family situations, where people don't want your success and are working against it. If certain members of your family are not who you would choose as friends, just love them but don't like them, and move on to a healthier situation for yourself.

This becomes even more complicated when this upwardly mobile situation leaves a spouse behind because they have not kept up their security. I have seen time and time again that the spouse that didn't get "the degree," was fine for the most part while the professional was getting the degree, because they could consider the professional a "student." However, when the professional got the diploma, then the other spouse's insecurities really came to the forefront and much drama ensued. Couples therapy is really important at this time. Individual therapy as well for the insecure spouse can be useful as long as this underlying causality is addressed right up front. The insecure spouse usually needs to understand their own self worth within their given talents. They also need to pursue goals they feel they may have missed, but this is usually not it. As a person, they need to understand a degree does not make the degree holder suddenly look down on people or see them as inferior. Someone can only be inferior to someone else with their permission, because they are insecure at a basic level about their own character. The insecure person can work on their character without ever getting a degree. Most people do. To try to make a degreed person miserable because it makes them feel a little better, somehow, dictates it is time to go to character school, or therapy or which ever of the two is most readily available in their area. It usually is very helpful for the other spouse to get counseling as well. It helps everyone to gain perspective on the dynamics at play and how to handle them.

At times people in a family, who feel left behind when another family member becomes upwardly mobile, project or "put on" the degreed person their own behavior that is the result of a lack of sophistication. Since they feel inadequate they usually project that the degreed person is being "controlling" or some such thing. This is invariably because the degreed person can approach a problem solving and planning issue from many more angles, due to their advanced education. The more insecure and unsophisticated the non-degreed family member is, the more threatened they will be by the family member who has more to offer in terms of ideas or solutions.

# CHAPTER TEN

## Not Everything is Dementia

---

### Coin #18:
Many conditions look like Dementia.

### Flip side:
Accurate diagnosis alleviates suffering.

### Coin #19:
People with Dementia can be in danger
of being taken advantage of.

### Flip side:
Prepare well for your final days and
surround yourself with caring people.

In the previous chapter I discuss unsophisticated family vs. more educated family members and the problems that can arise from this dichotomy. A lack of sophistication or education about the aged can also cause a lot of heartache and problems. Since psychiatrists go to school for an additional four years after medical school just to study Psychiatry, they get to know more about the nuances or unique presentations of more than just the most common presenting psychiatric conditions of the elderly. I once had someone tell me, "Well, if a doctor catches 80% of everything that's a B and that's pretty good." I was appalled. For the people who are in the other 20% it is a 100% missed diagnosis for them and can be a life sentence of misery.

There is something called Pseudodementia. This is a condition where older people seem demented or to be losing their faculties and memory. What really is happening is they are depressed. Depression in the elderly can mimic Dementia. Sometimes treating the depression alone can alleviate the symptoms. Often the elderly will only need a small amount of an antidepressant. This is because their functioning organs are older and are not working at full capacity, so a little goes a longer way. Remember that in a previous chapter I address that it takes some time for the nervous system to show improvement when treated, even thirty days as usual, at the right dose of medication. Sometimes it takes several weeks to get to the right dose. Don't give up on this treatment if the elderly person is depressed. If the depression is not treated and people just focus on, "Oh, it must be Dementia," you do a terrible disservice to the patient.

Sometimes a patient has both Dementia and Depression and both need to be treated. Usually you treat the Depression first to see what is remaining in the way of Dementia symptoms. Then you can treat the Dementia with the prevailing treatments as well.

Today we have medications that can help Dementia symptoms and seem to slow the progression of symptoms, when the elderly are treated early in the illness. It is good to get an evaluation at the first signs of memory problems. This is because the quality of life can be improved and a longer more enjoyable life can be the result.

Alzheimer's Dementia can start in the 50's and a certain type of forgetfulness is seen with this. Often this type of Dementia is intermittent. The patient may be fine for a period of time and then have a flare up of memory dysfunction, until it progresses.

There is a Dementia called Senile Dementia. This is usually seen in much later life and is more of a progressive, persistent type of elderly Dementia.

Sometimes the elderly get confused when they have not been eating properly. When their electrolytes are imbalanced they present as demented. Electrolytes are things like sodium and chloride and potassium. Many elderly patients are on medications that deplete their potassium. Many elderly are on sodium chloride restricted diets or they are just not eating enough to get the sodium chloride (salt) they actually need to think clearly. When the nutrition is improved and the electrolytes balanced, there can be a remarkable change for the better in mental status.

Dehydration can also cause confusion in the elderly. Sometimes it is hard to get the elderly to drink enough fluids, and it is hard for them to ambulate to the rest room so they decide to decrease their fluids to avoid having to get up and go to the bathroom. In some cases, they are demented as well and this compounds their cooperation and reasoning to hydrate properly. They are confused from Dementia and they worsen the confusion with dehydration. Hydrating with fluids can help the confusion from dehydration.

It is a good idea to consider multiple etiology in the presentation of the confused elderly. The confused elderly can have different combinations of problems on different days depending on the underlying causes of that day. The treatments should be tailored to the causes.

There also can be a loss of mental functioning due to various forms of space occupying lesions or brain tumors. This is not to be confused with Dementia. The reason this is so disastrous is that, of course, the treatment would be so different for the two conditions.

Today there are so many ways to treat brain tumors, cancerous and non-cancerous, with and without surgery, that assuming someone's mental decline is Dementia and not availing that person to a full medical workup by a brain specialist, is of course, unconscionable.

I know of one horrific situation where someone's relative was sequestered in a nursing home away from family and friends due to an estate conspiracy. All involved wished to call the elderly person's diagnosis, even in court documents, Dementia. The elderly person, however, off and on had had a meningioma. A meningioma is a benign brain tumor that had been previously operated on to relieve the potential of blindness, paralysis, etc. This operation had been performed decades before, with success. It was confirmed this meningioma had returned; yet even medical personal and others with advanced degrees, albeit not brain specialists, persisted in calling it Dementia. The elderly person proceeded, in isolation, to go partially blind, deaf, partially paralyzed, lose control of her abilities to use the restroom, etc. A neurologist was consulted by a concerned individual and it was confirmed that brain tumors can present "as if Dementia." Appeals were made to try to help this individual and were met with ferocious resistance. Was it ignorance by non-specialized medical personnel, the unsophisticated or otherwise intentioned family who had control of her estate, the untrained or blind trust in the available general medical doctor by the legal profession or other factors that allowed this individual to suffer so, at her last days, so needlessly? All because a diagnosis of "Dementia" persisted? Not everything is dementia. It can be other things. It can be other things that can be treated for a better quality life and it can be those things and Dementia in combination. Regardless, it is important to make the necessary distinctions for the dignity that our elderly deserve to the very end.

Dementia can be a serious time of life when certain types of people will not understand the condition and abuse the elderly or they will recognize their decline and abuse them by trying to take advantage of them.

Instances of ignorance can take the form of an attorney yelling abusively at them, or staff doing so at nursing homes, as they are frustrated and unschooled in the elderly ways.

Instances of victimization I was made aware of included a situation where an elderly man bought a $20,000.00 boat. His daughter told him he couldn't handle it so she sold it a few weeks later to her boyfriend for $7,000.00. The same man was taken to another state and put in a nursing home. This was after he was told he was to "take what he could grab and go" from the $100,000.00 addition he put on his daughter's home, to live out his life, after a fist fight with her over wanting to see his checkbook.

Since we are discussing the elderly I would like to discuss my philosophy of having the elderly enjoy their last days as much as possible.

Recently it has come to my attention that there are two theories about the end of people's lives.

My theory is that people should enjoy their life, all phases, as much as possible and this would include the end of their lives. I think that people have worked and earned through their lives to reap the rewards of enjoying what they have accomplished when they retire. I believe their children should help them in their old age and support their plans and desires and needs.

Apparently, some children feel entitled to the gains of the parents and their personal retirement. Instead of these grown children making their own way in life they look to the parents for total support or supplements of income. I know of so many cases of this. In one particular instance the more the parents were generous the more the adult children were hostile and talked badly of their parents to others and in a bullying way to their parents, too. The parents tried to appease the aggressive children but it ultimately ended up with a parent being abandoned in a nursing home, unvisited, with no pictures on the walls she could look at for orientation or comfort, no TV, no radio, no access to snacks, no telephone, no books or anyone to read to her or comfort her or give her news about those she had sacrificed for all her life. She was in a condition with only a few fake flowers, a small stuffed kitten, and a four dollar blanket, all thrown behind a curtain at the end of her bed in a two person room where she didn't even rate the window side. She was found screaming about being cold. She wanted chocolate for a milkshake that the med nurse gave her only a few sips of. Though she drank quite hungrily of the strawberry shake given her, she was left in her emaciated state, without even further strawberry sustenance, much less the chocolate that could have given her a little joy. She revealed to her visitor that she hid a tiny piece of color she looked at when things got really depressing for her. She was surviving in captivity. In America. In our nursing home system, at the hands of the children she never dreamed would decide this should be her final fate, when they got the Power of Attorney for her care. The social worker that witnessed this said that finding someone uncared for like this in a nursing home usually spoke to neglect by the local family. A caring daughter lived many miles away and was willing to devote time and travel to comfort and care for this relative but the local relatives went to great lengths to make sure this did not happen. It appeared this elderly woman could not die fast enough for the local children, who also saw to it that all of her personal effects were taken exclusively by them as if she were already dead.

I believe it would be easy for caring family or service organizations to brighten the days of our elderly. It can be done with small things, even just a visit.

I am a proponent of the drop in visit to nursing homes much the same way parents are told to do so at day care centers.

I am also someone who suggests the elderly take a very clear, serious look at to whom and when they give a Power of Attorney to, when and where they go to assisted living/ independent living arrangements, the reputation of the facilities, etc. It is best to clearly write out what you would like for the end of your life in as much detail as possible.

You should then have this notarized. This means you take it to your bank where they have a notary or to another notary and they affirm that you are signing it and put a seal on it. Then you need to keep it and copies of it in several safe places with several people you trust. You can keep it in a safety deposit box as long as someone you trust has the key if something happens to you, or be sure the key can be found in your effects.

Most of the time people give the Power of Attorney to children or relatives who live nearest to them or who have the most time to help them. Usually this makes sense. However, it is better to scrutinize the history of these relationships. It is best not to give the Power of Attorney to children who have a history of verbal and/or physical abuse towards you or other family members. Their problem will only become more magnified and they will escalate when you become feebler and more easily victimized. The

children described in the vignette above
included a local daughter who had been
turned down by her Korean pastor's wife
for a letter of recommendation to adopt
Korean children because of witnessing how
abusive she was. This same daughter never
had anything loving or kind to say about
her parents, or any successful relative, to
her other siblings. This daughter always
commented that the parents birthday and
holiday gifts were never enough, etc. When
her parents became vulnerable she and
her husband seized the opportunity to cut
out other sisters from the estate and more
importantly to further disadvantage and
disregard the parents in their greatest time
of need and protection, by influencing and
setting up barriers of access and other forms
of care. A kind sister went to this sister and
gently tried to approach her saying wouldn't
it be in the best interest for all that all the
sisters be involved in the care of their parents
at this important time in the parent's lives

The sister cruelly laughed and said a loud no and that she planned to ruin that particular sister's life and she had the council of her church to do so. Of course her particular brand of church had rationalized and stood to gain substantially financially from their misguided "Christian" deeds. Likely, all the history of this should be examined before giving your Power of Attorney over to such an individual, to care for you and make decisions for you, when you are in a feeble condition.

It is very important to have the right people surround you when you become incapacitated or demented. Plan for this way before it happens. If someone in your environment seems unsuitable in character, plan that this will get worse, not better as you become more vulnerable. Make arrangements for the best people, near or far, to have the power to make decisions for you, that you have clearly listed out and have put it in several accessible trusted places.

As you get older keep your depressions treated. Make sure you stay hydrated with fluids. Follow your salt restricted diet but if confusion sets in have your electrolytes tested and your salt intake adjusted as needed. Eat properly regardless of your age to avoid dietary confusions that could appear as Dementia or psychiatric conditions. Brain tumors deserve ongoing medical specialist evaluations and treatments, regardless of age.

# CHAPTER ELEVEN

## Don't Dismiss the Herbals

---

### Coin #20:
Fish oil capsules can help
psychiatric conditions.

### Flip side:
Vitamin E can help tremors, impotence,
and Tardive Dyskinesia.

### Coin #21:
Ginko Biloba seems to help memory.

### Flip side:
Melatonin helps sleep without
disturbing the dream cycle.

Vitamin therapy and herbals used to be in the realm of the hokey and laughable. Today bona fide well-respected research is being done on these supplements that can help mental illness.

Fish oil capsules or Omega-3 fatty acids, at about 1000 mg dose, has been used for many conditions. It has been researched and used to lower cholesterol, lower triglycerides, help inflammation, decrease skin wrinkles, etc. It has also been studied in pregnant women with Bipolar Disorder/Manic Depression, and studied in Depression. It is unusual to study anything in pregnant women due to the risks to mother and child. So, this type of study makes us take notice. Researchers think it helped some to alleviate the symptoms. The theory touted is that with the lives we live today (stress, fast food, etc.) our systems get an imbalance of Omega-3 fatty acids to the Omega-6 fatty acids and it is this imbalance that can actually cause a certain kind of Depression or depressive symptoms. Unless someone is taking a cholesterol lowering medication they can often be put on 1000 mg of Omega-3 fatty acids as an adjunct to their psychiatric medications, or in instances where they can't take medications for a while. This, of course, should be done with the advice of your doctor, as there may be other reasons you cannot take fish oil capsules or the doctor does not want you to. If you are allergic to fish you should not take fish oil capsules. Instead, you may be able to take flax seed for your Omega-3 fatty acids. You should not take flax seed if you are allergic to it or if there is a contraindication to it for any condition. Ask your doctor first.

If you take fish oil capsules, make sure they are mercury free. Some people have indigestion and there is a "burp-free" form of fish oil capsules that can be taken for a few dollars more.

Doses of up to four grams a day can be taken with fish oil capsules. This dosage and the titration of the dosage should be done with your doctor as many factors with herbals and vitamins make self-prescribing dangerous.

Vitamin E is used for several things in psychiatry. It is well researched for tremors of certain types and for side effects of muscle movements called Tardive Dyskinesia. The dosage of this should be left to your doctor. I read that the body only absorbs 200 IU of Vitamin E at a time so this could be considered when dosing. Vitamin E also thins the blood. Vitamin E can cause bruising and bleeding, especially if added to other things you are taking for blood thinning, such as aspirin. Before surgery, you should tell your doctor if you are on this vitamin, as often they will want you to discontinue it for a few days before a surgical procedure.

Sometimes Vitamin E is used when men

complain of impotence. The theory is likely that it does thin the blood and helps blood flow, and/or it does other things. Reports in practice are that it can help, even at 200 IU once a day.

Ginko Biloba, too, is supposed to thin the blood somewhat. It primarily was touted as helping memory, but studies recently say it doesn't help that. What I know is what I see in my practice. I get phone calls from nursing homes exclaiming the improvement in memory when people take even 60 mg. Once again, there are several dosages of this compound and your doctor is the best one to decide what, if any, you should try and for what reason. I don't claim here that it helps everyone with memory. There are so many causes of memory decline, and it has seemed to help some who have tried it for certain types of memory loss. The research and ultimate answers to its validity are ongoing, and memory loss can progress.

Melatonin is a good product for certain types of insomnia and shift sleep changes. It comes in a tablet form you swallow or an under the tongue form called "sublingual."

What is nice about the sublingual form is that when taken it hits the blood stream quickly and the patient falls asleep more reliably and quickly. The swallowed pill form takes at least fifteen minutes to get to the stomach and dissolve into the blood stream, etc. It is best when using the sublingual melatonin to already be in bed and ready to sleep when you put it under your tongue.

With melatonin there are several dosages. I usually recommend the 1mg sublingual size. The higher dosages usually are not "more is better." They seem to be too much and pop the patient awake after a few hours instead of getting the patient to sleep and keeping the patient asleep for a normal sleep cycle.

Speaking of normal sleep cycles, it is important when taking medications for sleep, that sleep cycles are considered. There are very few medications for sleep that do not disturb the normal sleep cycles and particularly, your REM sleep. REM sleep is where you dream and deal with the days events and disturbances. If you take sleeping pills for a long time and you don't get your proper REM sleep, this is not so good for you. If you are having trouble sleeping, it is usually best to find the underlying cause and treat that. Then, use your sleeping pills only short term. This is what they are devised for, until the underlying cause can be treated. If you are not sleeping because you are Bipolar, then treat your Bipolar Disorder with Bipolar medications, until you sleep properly. If you are depressed, and this is why you are not sleeping, then treat the Depression with the appropriate antidepressants until you sleep. This way your REM sleep will be intact and you won't need an additional sleeping pill.

Melatonin does not usually disturb the REM sleep and is used for occasional insomnia, for travel time change insomnia and when shift workers need to sleep at unusual times. Melatonin is a more natural substance that is even made in our systems when we are exposed to light. When we take it as a pill form it is being introduced into our systems as if we are getting a bump of it like we are exposed to light. This is how it helps travelers and shift workers sleep at times they don't ordinarily do so. Some research shows that it helps to take melatonin before ten o'clock at night for best results, and sometimes, researchers also suggest starting at lower than 1 mg to start. Melatonin is contraindicated in Diabetes. You should always check with your doctor before taking melatonin, or any vitamin or herbal for whatever reason.

# CHAPTER TWELVE

## Weight Loss Tips

---

### Coin #22:
Walking is the secret weight loss tip you always pay for in the magazines.

### Flip side:
Find an activity you like to do or chain movement to something you like to do.

### Coin #23:
Keep a food diary.

### Flip side:
Add things to lose weight.

Almost every magazine at the supermarket touts that they have a great idea for weight loss. Once you spend the money it almost always says: "MOVE MORE AND EAT LESS." Then they say all the research shows that walking produces the best results. They usually discuss that our bodies were made to walk and burn calories this way and this activity perfectly dove tails to our needing to take in calories when we eat. Europeans walk a great deal. They also seem to eat a great deal. For the most part, Europeans seem to be more fit.

Few people in America walk. There are things that could make it easier to do this along with other activities.

## TO MOVE MORE:

1. Try parking your car a little further from the door at work each day. You could also do this shopping. You will expend a few

more calories walking a little further, which the magazines all say is the perfect exercise for us and gets the best results. Walking is also free. It doesn't require a lot of extra equipment or memberships.

2. On the days it is raining or too cold to park further away, substitute stair walking more than you usually do. Any extra you do will be calories burned.

3. Get a pedometer at any sporting goods store and make a GOAL/REWARD/PLAN for increasing the number of steps to the car or on the stairs you complete. Reward yourself with anything but food or alcohol for increased steps. It could be a download of a new song or an extra long bubble bath, or donate something to a special cause that makes you feel wonderful (this can be expanded on to where you put away a dollar for reaching a certain increase in steps every day and then each month you have that great

feeling of donating the total at your favorite charity), get a pedicure or manicure, golf an extra day or another nine holes, buy yourself special sporting event tickets, etc.

There are ways of setting up a reward system where you can see your progress. You can tangibly put away a quarter or dollar in a jar for accomplishment per day, then just go spend it on what you what. This cements that you are rewarding yourself for progress. This is important one way or another. Many people get the reward feedback with the results of fitness or weight loss. Most of the time though, being human beings, people need something tangible to keep up the encouragement. Humans need positive reinforcement and reward. Just make sure the reward is a healthy reward that cements your gains in a positive way.

4. Do an ACTIVITY you like and don't call it exercise. Most exercise routines last two

weeks because the brain views this as torture. If you like to dance, take dance lessons or go to dance clubs. If you like to hike, hike. If you like to try new things look into scuba lessons or repelling on the fake mountain at the sporting goods store or golf lessons or sailing, etc. Join a volleyball or bowling league.

5. Chain, or attach, walking, in your neighborhood, to something else that is enjoyable, like listening to really good music with headphones, or recorded books you can rent from the library. Make your phone calls via Bluetooth as you walk and multitask. Swim with the news on or a movie, so you "kill two birds with one stone" and catch up on your media at the same time. Watch TV or a movie on your cell phone.

6. DON'T THINK/DO. Usually we spend so much time thinking about if we feel like exercising or "do we want to," that if we

had just done something during that time we would be way ahead of the exercise, or I mean, ACTIVITY game.

7.  Do something you enjoy, that you see as activity, not exercise, or chain something enjoyable to exercise, and just do it without thinking, Have a back up for when you can't do your usual routine (if the weather is bad or you are on vacation, etc).

8.  Use barbells or that treadmill you bought, during commercials while watching TV. A study I read showed that women lost several more pounds a month when they broke up their exercise into ten minutes four times a day. This would make some sense as women are different from men and our activity is usually more in spurts, as when you look way back in caveman history with child rearing. The studies that ask for 20 to 30 minutes a day of exercise from people were almost always done with men.

9. I usually suggest that people start with five minutes for the activity they have chosen. Starting with thirty minutes is daunting. If you start with five minutes you feel success. When you find you overshoot five minutes, easily, then do ten minutes. Once you condition you will find you accidentally did fifteen minutes, easily. Now you can do fifteen minutes, and so on.

10.    Don't have any excuses. There are so many things listed above and so many more you can think of that there just are not any excuses for not moving more and enjoying it!

## TO LOSE WEIGHT:

1. Don't drop below 1500 calories for women or 2000 calories for guys in a given 24 hours. You will lose just as much weight with these calories as the lower ones and you will be able to sustain your diet plan. You want to have a lifetime plan. If you go

to the really lower calorie plans it resets your brain and then later, when you must eat more, your body sees it as something to store and you gain weight back. If you eat fewer calories than you have been, then you will lose. You also can eat too few calories to lose weight. If you have been eating too few calories you haven't anything to fuel and burn what calories you are getting.

2. Keep a food diary for a week. This is usually eye opening. When you add up the calories you will see if you are getting too few or too many. You can also see where the fast food is coming in, the secret eating, the samples at the supermarket, the extra cookie, the denial eating that, oops, adds up.

3. Look at your food diary and see if there is anything you can swap out for a lower calorie item. Don't deprive yourself. Eat things you like or you will never be successful long term. However, there may be some things

you can substitute for high calorie stuff that are just as good and you will never miss the original. For instance, there is a brand of soy cheese in every flavor that is low fat and no cholesterol. Use that on sandwiches and you would never miss the calories or the taste of the higher fat version.

4. Eliminate one thing you wouldn't really mind. I know one lady who stopped getting her fountain drinks and she lost 70 pounds in one year. She did nothing else to change her diet.

5. If your appetite says "hungry" all the time, consider that you might be one of the people sensitive to high fructose corn syrup. There is some controversy about this but it seems to help some people to eliminate it from their diet. It seems to take three days after their last encounter with it, and then they just don't have the constant food drive to eat. After a three-day clean out of high fructose

corn syrup they say they feel satisfied on less food. Watch out for versions of this on the nutritional labels, though, such as "fructose" and "corn syrup solids," etc.

6. There is also some controversy about diet pop and preservatives and weight gain. Most people recommend eight, 8-ounce glasses of water a day as helpful to losing weight, and this seems well researched. It is on almost every diet plan and program out there.

7. I like adding things instead of deprivation:

Calcium seems to be well researched as helpful to weight loss.

Spices such as hot sauce and mustard seem to increase metabolism.

Matcha green tea, even the decaffeinated version, or four cups a day of white or green tea has been researched to increase metabolism, even decaf.

Cinnamon seems to help even blood sugars and was researched to help weight loss. A nice low calorie treat can be cinnamon toast made with a little melted butter and a sprinkling of a mixture together of 1 tsp of cinnamon and 1 tsp of low calorie sugar substitute.

8. Eating several small meals throughout the day keeps the metabolism from dropping and is even supposed to help speed it up.

9. Eating one large meal a day defeats several things. It messes with #8 above and #10 below.

10. Eat only when you are hungry and stop when you are full. You likely are metabolizing when you are hungry. When you eat past when you feel full, then what you eat is likely stored directly as fat.

11. Keep small sandwich bags of non-perishable low calorie treats in your car to keep from a whole meal stop at the drive in. This can be a handful of un-roasted almonds (not all the calories are absorbed from nuts), a hand full of crackers or grapes or anything that works for you.

12. Positive self-talk is essential for successful weight loss and maintenance. Much research went into the eating disorders of Anorexia Nervosa and Bulimia. The outshoots of this were that for these disorders and for overeating habits and weight loss the more positive a person's self-talk the more successful the individual was with their goals. Many times with these situations people develop a negative mantra in their heads about themselves and how they are eating/looking/exercising. This usually causes the situation to worsen and not improve. The more positive statements the person could go to about themselves for their efforts, the

less they fell back into negative toxic habits. Try a more positive spin on things. If you eat more than you planned, say to yourself, "Well, I didn't eat the whole package" or "In the old days I would have eaten two." Always remind yourself of the gains already made. Keep a journal of these to go to if it is hard to be positive on certain days and you feel you have slipped. Always immediately state a positive thought when a negative one creeps in to counter it. This is a good way to change the bad habit of negativity and soon mostly positive thoughts will prevail as you persist with this.

13. Regularity is very important. Constipation can best be dealt with by three or four glasses of water first thing in the morning. The products by prescription for irregularity sometimes are just pulling fluid from your body. It makes more sense to just add it directly to your gastrointestinal tract, by drinking water. It may take a few

days of this to improve things. Fiber is also very important. There are so many delicious whole grain things and fiber bars that are like candy bars now, that this can actually be a treat in your food plan.

14. Add more fruits and vegetables. I know this sounds trite. The deal is to find a couple of fruits you really like. Try some new ones. A serving is usually 1/2 cup so that is not so much. On most diet programs they say that if you need something more than what was allotted for the day, by way of their program, your safest thing is to add fruit. Fruit juices though, seem to add to weight gain when increased past one or two servings a day. Toss in a salad once in a while. Find a salad mix you like. Put it in a large sandwich bag, add a serving of dressing you like, close up the seal and shake until all the lettuce is covered. You can use way less of the dressing (a diet downfall) when you do this, as all the lettuce and other veggies in your salad get covered

with the dressing. Eat tomatoes like an apple. Add mustard or your hot sauce as a dip for your tomato. Try this with other vegetables. Be creative. Go down the fruit and vegetable aisles with new eyes and a fresh brain. Think out of the box, literally, when you venture down the fruit and vegetable aisles.

# CHAPTER THIRTEEN

## Educational Minutes

---

I have included a collection of instructional EDUCATIONAL MINUTES that aired on a radio station. When the station called me and asked me to do an interview, and then to record some instructional pieces, I thought these would be the most helpful.

# AN EDUCATIONAL MINUTE
# FROM DR. SHILLING: #1

---

**Coin #24:**
Seasonal Affective Disorder (SAD) is a
unique biochemical depression.

**Flip side:**
The wavelength of sunlight is the best
treatment for SAD.

---

Post holiday blues can be a biochemical
condition unique to winter. It is called
Seasonal Affective Disorder. This form of
depression and other serious depressions
can be treated. Your spiritual background
is an important strength to help improve
conditions when you work as a team with
a Psychiatrist. Depression can be a real
physical condition that should not be
ignored.

# AN EDUCATIONAL MINUTE
# FROM DR. SHILLING: #2

---

## Coin #25:
Psychiatrists are trained for many years just to treat mental illness.

## Flip side:
Some Mental Illness is physical like Diabetes or Thyroid Disease.

---

Many people do not know what a Psychiatrist is. Psychiatrists get an M.D. in medical school, then they go to school for another four years just to focus on psychiatric conditions. All this training is necessary to treat depressions, panic disorders and many other conditions that are on a physical basis, due to biochemical problems, as are Diabetes or Thyroid Disorders.

# AN EDUCATIONAL MINUTE
# FROM DR. SHILLING: #3

## Coin #26:
There are two types of depression.

## Flip side:
There are situational depressions and there are biochemical depressions.

Many people don't know there are two types of depression. There is Situational Depression and there is a more serious form of physical depression that is biochemical. Psychiatrists can diagnose and give specific treatments for both types of depressions.

# CHAPTER FOURTEEN

## Articles

**The following are a collection of articles written over the years for various newspapers.**

**The coins are placed before each article.**

There is a religious overtone to some of the articles as one of the papers that asked me to contribute was spiritual in nature. I share my Christian faith personally. Professionally, it is important for me to indicate that I see patients of all faiths and non-faiths and I enjoy this very much.

My faith is one of tolerance and kindness and a non-judgmental attitude. This is how I interpret the teachings of Christianity. I hope the readers of my book and articles come to opinions the same way and do not consider me to be of a lock-step nature in my opinions, or that I am in one particular box, because I hold certain beliefs.

I think one of the most important things in emotional and psychiatric growth is the sharing of ideas and beliefs. It is through our intellectual, spiritual and emotional pursuits that we can advance as a people whether we agree on all tenets or bases or none. It is through dialogue and differences we expand and learn, cement our own beliefs or change. It is all good, when viewed with the best attitude. It is my guess that everyone reading this book believes in something even if that something is nothing.

Enjoy my articles on the various subjects.

# ARTICLE #1
# HOLIDAY BLUES

---

**Coin #27:**
Holiday Depressions can have many causes.

**Flip side:**
Prioritize to make a happier holiday.

---

This isn't another article on the "holiday blues." The usual article gives you ten tips on how to handle stress or offers platitudes about family relationships.

Holiday Depression like many other depressions can be due to many causes.

Some people get more depressed in the winter and actually have a biochemical problem due to a lack of quality sunshine. This is often easily treated by a 10,000-

LUX sunlight replacement and/or newer biochemical specific medications.

Some Bipolar (Manic/Depression) conditions are subject to seasonal changes and medications may need to be temporarily adjusted.

Situational Depressions or Adjustment Disorders with Depression can be worsened by good or bad stress and situations of unique or unusual change. A Situational Depression can be in addition to a biochemical depression (Major Depression).

The holidays are all about changes. There are the changes of weather, the change of wardrobes, the change in foods, the change in family patterns, the change in time devoted to exercise, friends, and church activities, etc. Limit setting on many of these changes is only possible to a certain degree. Change is just a fact of life. The more flexible we can be the more we can withstand the negative side of change. Studies have shown that those who can adjust and bend to changes in their life seem to be healthier and live longer. Expecting change and planning for it can help diminish the negative impact of change. Preparation for change can include putting things aside to be done after the holidays, establishing unwavering priorities (devotions, exercise, church, etc), decreasing nonessential time consuming activities temporarily (TV, telephone calls, etc) and increasing organization (car pools, delegation tasks, etc).

One of the key things to helping holiday blues and the inevitable changes of the holidays is to harness perfectionist tendencies. The advertisements and commercials want us to believe that our homes should look perfect, our food should be ideal and homemade, and every one of our family relationships should be non-dysfunctional, if even for a little while. Setting our expectations too high for the holidays can ensure depression of some type. Life is imperfect and we are imperfect human beings. The adage of "doing the best you can do, what more can you do" is a good one to remember. Do your best but plan for imperfection. This realistic approach will help you enjoy all the special changes of the holidays as well as the difficulties. Decide what the most important things are to you at this time of the year and sift out the things that are not. When you have thought through a plan on how to handle seasonal changes there will be less guilt and depression about not doing everything or not doing everything perfectly. Some if not most of your holiday can be happy.

# ARTICLE #2
# HOW TO HELP STOP THE SHOOTERS

---

**Coin #28:**
We all need to help to stop mass shootings.

**Flip side:**
There are always options of help
for those who feel drastic.

---

In the wake of the recent mall and church shootings in our nation we all reflect on what more can be done to help the lost and hopeless who think such actions are the way to deal with their mental anguish and pain.

1. Take suicidal and homicidal threats seriously. Almost all who commit these acts give warning first.

2. Get psychiatric help for those who talk suicidal, homicidal or nonsensical disjointed speech.

Because of their illness they are hard to reason with, can be irrational and disorganized and need your help in getting to a psychiatrist or an ER even for an evaluation.

3. Go the extra mile.

Even though someone may have had treatment in the past, their condition could be chronic. This means they may need unflagging support to get yet more treatment, stay in treatment or stay on their medications.

4. Resist uninformed comments about psychiatric medications.

The       medications       for       psychiatric

conditions today are useful. These medications help neurochemistry that can be out of balance from genetic inherited conditions or extreme stress that is toxic to the brain. Psychiatric conditions are medical conditions the same as Diabetes or Thyroid Disorders, for instance.

Psychiatric medications aren't mood-altering drugs that will make someone be something other than their healthy self.

Do not tell someone on psychiatric meds that it is "time to stop or decrease their meds." This decision should be a medical one made by a doctor (Psychiatrist).

5. Avoid simplistic solutions for complex problems.

Often people with psychiatric conditions have multiple problems. They may have drug and alcohol problems as well as other psychiatric diagnoses (Bipolar Disorder, Schizophrenia, Multiple Personalities).

They will need AA as well as a Psychiatrist. Treating only one aspect of a condition will be inadequate.

Half-treated psychiatric conditions often lead patients to self medicate with street drugs and alcohol. Alcohol is liquid depression. Street drugs further imbalance neurochemicals. Alcohol and street drugs may make people feel better for a short time but the aftermath leaves people worse off neurochemcially.

6. Impress that there are always options.

People who have biochemical depressions often lose sight of options. They may think they only have one solution to their pain. They need to be reminded that there are always multiple options to problems.

7. Encourage people not to give up or "snap."

People in mental pain need to keep reaching out to doctors, therapists, clergy, hotlines, etc., until they get their relief by professionals. Drastic measures are not necessary to deal with life's most difficult times. Help is available. They can get through the worst time of their life to go on to happier times and a fulfilled life.

8. Be kinder.

The mentally ill are very sensitive to judgmental looks and attitudes towards those who sometimes seem out of place or different. Kindness and diplomacy should be easy. It could go a long way to help anyone in need of a little de-stressing. Kindness and caring will make our world a better place.

# ARTICLE #3
# BIBLE ONLY?

## Coin #29:
Some church people feel judged in their
church for having biochemical mental illness.

## Flip side:
Compassion, education, and spirituality
help treat mental illness.

What would Jesus do? So many times I have
had patients who say they feel condemned or
judged for suffering from mental illness or
taking psychotropic medications. It would be
unlikely that Jesus would do so. His example is
one of compassion. At the heart of the matter
is awareness. Many people do not understand
that certain depressions and other mental
illnesses are biochemical problems, much like
Diabetes or Thyroid Disease. When someone's

symptoms reach a certain degree they no longer are matters for simple solutions. A trained psychiatrist can decipher if a depression is just situational and treatable by simple means or more complex and a biochemical depression. A biochemical depression needs the spiritual attention but also the wonderful medical attention God has made available today. Researchers believe there are two main types of biochemical depression. One type is due to an imbalance of serotonin, a brain neurotransmitter. Another type of depression is thought to be primarily due to the imbalance of the brain neurotransmitter norepinephrine. The treatment is different for each type of depression and a medically trained psychiatrist can differentiate the type of depression and the appropriate treatment for it. Sometimes these depressions are genetic and as such are inherited through the genes. Sometimes these depressions are from an overload of stress that results in the biochemical imbalance. Whatever the reason for the depression, compassion and psychiatric help should be the focus of the church. After all, Christ would want us to follow his example. Since people are human and not capable of being God themselves they will suffer illness and the best way to fight it is with all of the God given talents and products he has put on earth. Help someone near or dear to you to feel comfortable about reaching out to get the help that is there. Don't be a stumbling block against someone reaching his or her full potential and abilities. Jesus would of course heal the sick as his many examples in the Bible show. Short of that miracle happening, why deny the chance at a more fulfilled life, utilizing their gifts, with the many treatments available, until such time as perfect healing could occur? This approach applies to other religions, not just Christianity, where it would be best for education and compassion and the tenets of kindness to prevail over ignorance and myths and judgment.

# ARTICLE #4
# HUMOR IS A GOOD
# DEFENSE MECHANISM

---

## Coin #30:
Humor is a good way to deal with problems.

## Flip side:
We need to use all types of treatments to help the many different problems and diagnoses.

---

A merry heart doeth good like a medicine (Prov. 17:22). What an important part of God's message. What an enlightenment and edification to our soul. Like everything else in the Bible, medical science has proven that humor and laughter are very healing vehicles. We would do better to bring more healthy laughter and merriment to our daily lives. Good wholesome fun. What an endowment from the Lord.

A lot of what science has found through research can be found originally in the Bible. This holds true for mental health. God charges us to rejoice, (2 Chr. 6, 41, 29, 27), to be of good cheer and to worship with merriment and song as each gift has been individually imparted to his flock. Sadness likewise is addressed in the scriptures (Mark 10, 22).

Routinely, scripture speaks to the situational forms of the emotions of sadness and happiness. Situational happiness or depression is that which is due to the situations we find our self in or seek out. But what of the sadness or excessive merriment conditions that are of a biochemical basis? I speak of the conditions that are due to a biochemical or neurotransmitter imbalance or genetic lack of production. St. Luke was a physician faced with these much deeper and non-situational conditions. He treated them the best he knew how with the then prevailing remedies. Throughout subsequent centuries the physicians treated with the latest treatment options available. What joy today that there are the types of treatment medications that seem to work at the cellular neurotransmitter level to help a person's natural biochemicals finally do the work God intended them to. What joy to hear patients say that they have a right sense of self, can pray again with meaning and fervor, can partake of the understanding of grace and can participate fully in service.

Often in my practice I try to bring humor to my psychotherapy and medication management sessions. This helps to alleviate, in therapeutic ways, the layer of situational things, so the deeper can be dealt with. Formal psychiatry has recognized humor as a "good defense mechanism." The Lord could have told them that long ago. Yes, humor is a superior way to deal with what the world gives us, the situational. It of course can help in the moderate and severe psychiatric conditions of the biochemical nature, too. Good cheer is so important to augment the heaven sent, neurologically specific medications, that work to bolster the patient's natural biochemicals, restoring someone to health. God's grace is truly seen in this.

Everyone who has situational ups or downs knows what a little good cheer can do. It is sometimes hard for us to understand what it would be like to have the more severe forms of a biochemical genetic ups and downs that can rob a person of their joy and ability to fully partake of cheer. When there is understanding, education and awareness of the different types of depression, someone can get proper diagnosis and treatment. Subsequently, individuals can be restored to where they again are able to partake of all of God's beauty. They once again can laugh in their situations, with their cheer passed on yet to heal others. Yes, a merry heart doeth good like medicine.

# NOTES

# NOTES

# NOTES

# NOTES

# NOTES

# NOTES

# NOTES